Mutagenesis and Mitochondrial-Associated Pathologies

Edited by Michael Fasullo and Angel Catala

Published in London, United Kingdom

Mutagenesis and Mitochondrial-Associated Pathologies
http://dx.doi.org/10.5772/intechopen.98146
Edited by Michael Fasullo and Angel Catala

Contributors
Lovelesh K. Kumar Nigam, Aruna V. Vanikar, Rashmi Dalsukhbhai Patel, Kamal V. Kanodia, Kamlesh Suthar, Umang Thakkar, Lata Singh, Mithalesh Kumar Singh, Sanket Tembe, Angel Catala, Christine Richardson, Kiran Lalwani, Caroline French, Boris Chadov, Nina Fedorova

First published in London, United Kingdom, 2022 by IntechOpen
IntechOpen is the global imprint of INTECHOPEN LIMITED, registered in England and Wales, registration number: 11086078, 5 Princes Gate Court, London, SW7 2QJ, United Kingdom

British Library Cataloguing-in-Publication Data
A catalogue record for this book is available from the British Library

Additional hard and PDF copies can be obtained from orders@intechopen.com

Mutagenesis and Mitochondrial-Associated Pathologies
Edited by Michael Fasullo and Angel Catala
p. cm.
Print ISBN 978-1-80355-171-5
Online ISBN 978-1-80355-172-2
eBook (PDF) ISBN 978-1-80355-173-9

For EU product safety concerns:
IN TECH d.o.o., Prolaz Marije Krucifikse Kozulić 3, 51000 Rijeka, Croatia,
info@intechopen.com or visit our website at intechopen.com.

Meet the editors

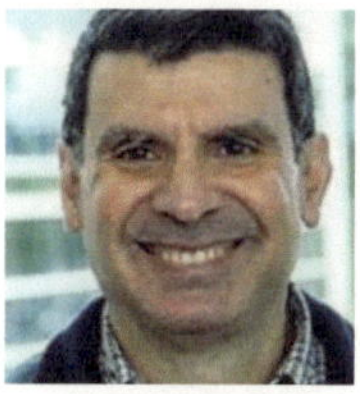

Michael Fasullo, Ph.D., is an associate professor at SUNY Polytechnic University, New York. He earned a BSc at the Massachusetts Institute of Technology and a Ph.D. at the Department of Biochemistry, Stanford University, California. He was an American Cancer Society fellow at Columbia University, New York, and held faculty positions at Loyola University Chicago and Albany Medical College, New York. He has authored more than forty peer-reviewed publications, book chapters, and review articles in the field of yeast genetics, DNA recombination and repair, oncolytic viruses, and toxicology. His present work focuses on profiling the yeast and mammalian genome for resistance to P450-activated mycotoxins and heterocyclic amines. His research has been funded by the National Institutes of Health, Department of Defense, March of Dimes, and Leukemia Research Foundation.

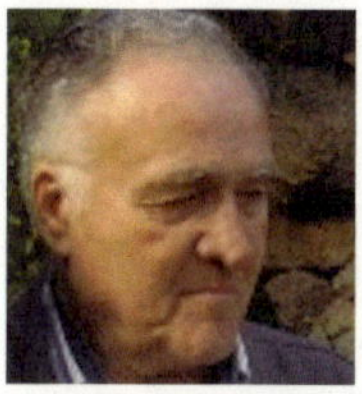

Angel Catalá studied chemistry at Universidad Nacional de La Plata, Argentina, where he received a Ph.D. in Chemistry (Biological Branch) in 1965. From 1964 to 1974, he worked as an Assistant in Biochemistry at the School of Medicine at the same university. From 1974 to 1976, he was a fellow of the National Institutes of Health (NIH) at the University of Connecticut, Health Center, USA. From 1985 to 2004, he served as a Full Professor of Biochemistry at the Universidad Nacional de La Plata. He is a member of the National Research Council (CONICET), Argentina, and the Argentine Society for Biochemistry and Molecular Biology (SAIB). His laboratory has been interested for many years in the lipid peroxidation of biological membranes from various tissues and different species. Dr. Catalá has directed twelve doctoral theses, published more than 100 papers in peer-reviewed journals, several chapters in books, and edited twelve books. He received awards at the 40th International Conference Biochemistry of Lipids 1999 in Dijon, France. He is the winner of the Bimbo Pan-American Nutrition, Food Science and Technology Award 2006 and 2012, South America, Human Nutrition, Professional Category. In 2006, he won the Bernardo Houssay award in pharmacology, in recognition of his meritorious works of research. Dr. Catalá belongs to the editorial board of several journals including *Journal of Lipids; International Review of Biophysical Chemistry; Frontiers in Membrane Physiology and Biophysics; World Journal of Experimental Medicine and Biochemistry Research International; World Journal of Biological Chemistry, Diabetes, and the Pancreas; International Journal of Chronic Diseases & Therapy;* and *International Journal of Nutrition*. He is the co-editor of *The Open Biology Journal* and associate editor for *Oxidative Medicine and Cellular Longevity*.

Contents

Preface

Reactive oxygen species (ROS) and DNA double-strand breaks have been associated with multiple clinical pathologies and genetic mutations. Increased levels of ROS have been associated with cancer progression, Alzheimer's disease, and cardiovascular diseases. Dysfunctional mitochondria can internally generate ROS, resulting in increased Ca++ flux, inflammation, or apoptosis. ROS is also generated by exposure to external environmental factors, including ionizing radiation, industrial toxicants, and food carcinogens. ROS-induced germline and stem cell mutations can lead to developmental deformities. Our continual exposure to ROS underscores the urgency to understand how ROS-associated DNA damage can be repaired, recognize ROS-associated pathologies, and find cures for diseases that result from dysfunctional mitochondria.

Recently, gene therapy has shown promise for the treatment of inherited diseases, such as sickle cell disease. Much of this success can be credited to advances in gene editing techniques, notably CRISPR/CAS9, and in the utilization of model animal organisms, such as mice. The success of CRISPR/CAS9 in editing nuclear genes has excited interest in editing mitochondrial genomes. However, editing mitochondria genes is challenging, partially due to the need to permeate both the outer and inner membranes. In addition, some cells exhibit mitochondrial heteroplasmy. Alternative possibilities are also being explored, such as the ablation of the mutated mitochondrial genome and mitochondrial transplantation.

The chapters in this book highlight pathologies that result from mitochondrial dysfunction and mutagenesis that results from double-strand breaks. The first section focuses on mitochondrial diseases with chapters on ocular and renal pathologies and emerging genetic editing strategies to mitigate or correct mitochondrial DNA mutations. The second section focuses on model organisms and mutagenesis. Of particular interest are transgenic mouse models followed by a chapter on the identification of radiation-induced ontogenic mutations in Drosophila. Altogether, these chapters provide novel insights into mitochondrial-associated diseases and experimental model organisms to study the repair and consequences of DNA damage.

Michael Fasullo
College of Nanoscale Science and Engineering,
SUNY Polytechnic Institute,
Albany, New York, United States

Angel Catala
Facultad de Ciencias Exactas,
Instituto de Investigaciones Fisicoquímicas Teóricas y Aplicadas (INIFTA-CCT La Plata-CONICET),
Universidad Nacional de La Plata,
La Plata, Argentina

Section 1

Mitochondrial Diseases

Chapter 1

Introductory Chapter: Mitochondrial Diseases - Advances and Perspectives - My Point of View

Angel Catala

1. Introduction

There is only one metabolic pathway that is under the dual control of the mitochondrial genome (mtDNA) and the nuclear genome (nDNA). Disorders in the mitochondrial respiratory chain are called by convention "mitochondrial diseases." Mitochondrial disorders symbolize a major challenge in medicine. Much of the mitochondrial proteins are encoded by nuclear DNA (nDNA), while only a few are encoded by mitochondrial DNA (mtDNA). Mutations in mtDNA or mitochondrial-related nDNA genes can cause a mitochondrial disorder. The disorder can affect multiple organs in different locations and severity; but there are some ways that involve only one organ. Modifications of the mitochondrial oxidative phosphorylation system can generate mutations in both mitochondrial DNA and nuclear DNA that lead to mitochondrial diseases. Mitochondrial diseases comprise a diverse group of genetic disorders, which appear at any age and have a wide spectrum of clinical symptoms. This leads to highly changeable cases, making it difficult to diagnose mitochondrial diseases. The latest advances in genetic testing and original reproductive options hold great promise for improving the clinical recognition and treatment of mitochondrial diseases. In this chapter we discuss developments in the recognition and diagnosis of mitochondrial diseases. In the last five decades, the effect of mitochondrial diseases on biological systems began to be widely investigated. This chapter explains the most important aspects in our opinion of mitochondrial diseases.

2. Brief history of mitochondria

The generation of adenosine triphosphate by oxidative phosphorylation occurs in the mitochondria; about 90% of the cell's energy need is satisfied during the hydrolysis of ATP produced in this way. In addition, mitochondria are also involved in other processes including, but not limited to, the formation of iron and sulfur groups, the citric acid cycle, the regulation of apoptosis1, and calcium homeostasis in conjunction with the endoplasmic reticulum.

Mitochondria do not have nearly the amount of DNA necessary to encode all the specific proteins of mitochondria; however, millions of years of evolution could explain a progressive loss of autonomy. The endosymbiotic hypothesis could be called a theory, but no experimental reason can be offered to test it. Only indirect confirmation can be accessed in support of the proposal, which is the most likely justification for the mitochondria starting point. The verification necessary to change the model from hypothesis to theory is probably forever lacking in ancient times.

3. Mitochondrial diseases

Studies of genetic pathologies that affect mitochondrial metabolism as a consequence of modifications in genes encoded by mitochondrial DNA or genes encoded by nuclear DNA for dynamic proteins inside the mitochondria began in 1988. Since that year, a new notional "mitochondrial genetics" has become visible; based on three attributes of mtDNA: (1) polyplasmy; (2) maternal inheritance; and (3) mitotic segregation. Diagnosis of mtDNA-connected diseases was completed through genetic analysis and experimental advances that incorporated histochemical staining of muscle or brain sections, single-fiber polymerase chain reaction (PCR) of mtDNA, and the design of a "hybrid" Immortal (cytoplasmic hybrid) derivative from patient fibroblast cell lines.

4. My participation in studies with mitochondria

In the last three decades, our laboratory has investigated the lipid peroxidation of biological membranes of various tissues and different species, as well as liposomes prepared with phospholipids with a high content of polyunsaturated fatty acids. We analyzed the effect of various antioxidants such as alpha tocopherol, vitamin A, melatonin and its structural analogues and conjugated linoleic acid, among others [1, 2]. The integrity of the mitochondrial membranes and the function of numerous protein complexes in the ETC [3] are determined by cardiolipin, which is a unique class of specific mitochondrial phospholipids that exist almost exclusively in the inner membrane of mitochondria (IMM). In most mammalian tissues, tetralinoleoylcardiolipin (L4CL) is the main form of cardiolipins, this molecule contains four chains of structural linoleic acid. The incorporation of four LA side chains into L4CL and their presence in mitochondria allow L4CL to be easily oxidized by reactive oxygen species and then to generate an electrophilic reaction **Figure 1** [4].

5. Conclusions

Aging and age-related diseases have been connected with mitochondrial uncoupling and elevated ROS formation. Dysfunctional mitochondria incline to modified lipid metabolism and augmented lipid peroxidation products. Mitochondrial antioxidants that can re-establish function and prevent pathological lipid peroxidation are showing guarantee in diminishing biological aging and therefore they may offer advantage for slowing the development to age-related diseases such as neurodegeneration. In parallel, novel drug groups are providing a unusual strategy to delay aging during elimination of senescent cells. By mean of these drugs as instruments offer a chance to amplify our understanding of whether the alterations in reactive oxygen species, lipid metabolism and mitochondrial lipids detected during aging and diseases are due to the increase of senescent cells.

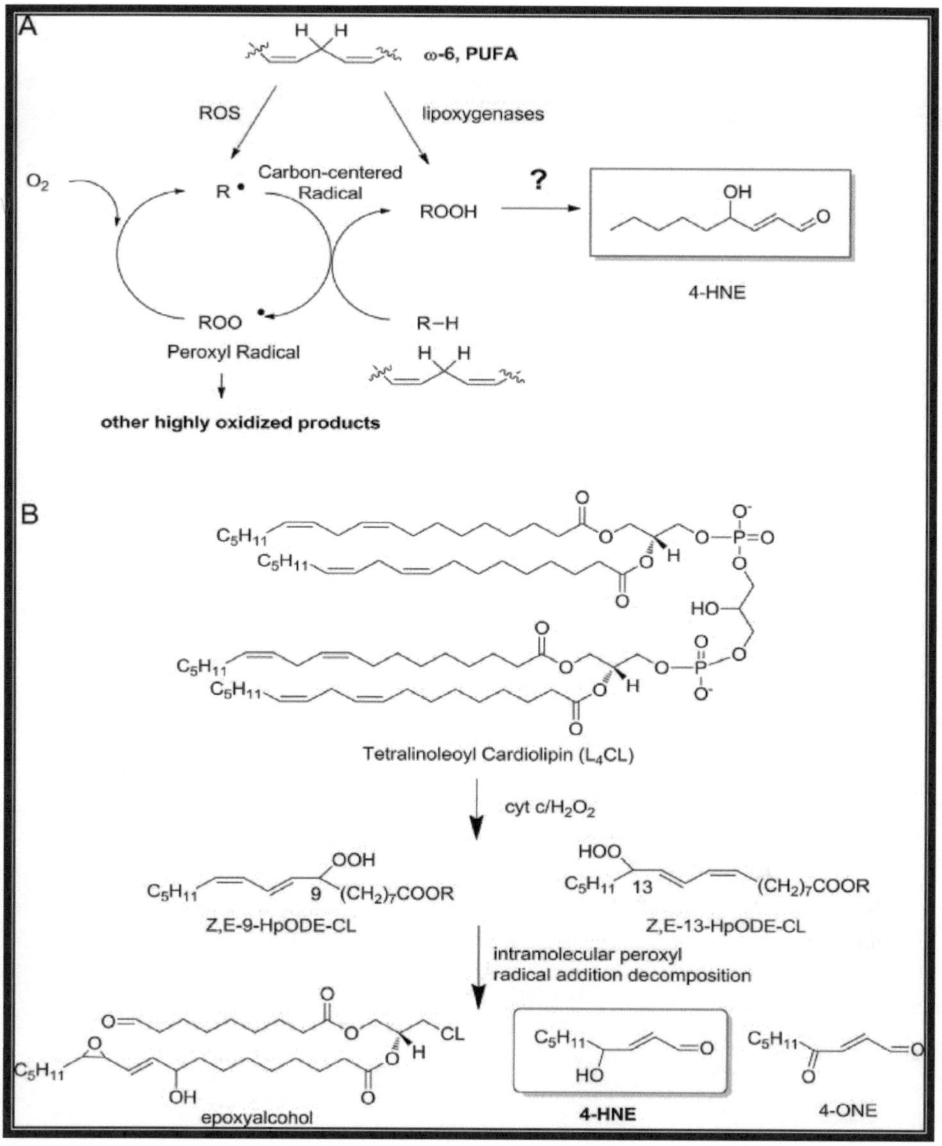

Figure 1.
Chemical mechanisms for 4-HNE formation from lipid peroxidation. (A) General scheme for the formation of 4-HNE from decomposition of lipid hydroperoxides that can be generated from free radical oxidation of ω-6 PUFA or enzymatic oxidation by lipoxygenases. (B) Lipid electrophiles generated from oxidation of mitochondrial cardiolipin: Oxidation of L_4CL by the peroxidase activity of cyt c and CL complex in the presence of H_2O_2 results in the formation of hydroperoxyoctadecadienoic acid (HpODE), 9-HpODE-CL and 13-HpODE-CL. During this process, through intra-molecular peroxyl radical addition and decomposition of an unstable intermediate, several reactive aldehydes are produced including epoxyalcohol-aldehyde-CL (EAA-CL), 4-HNE, and 4-oxo-2-nonenal (4-ONE). Reproduced from Redox Biol. 2015 Apr; 4: 193–199. Rights Managed by Elsevier.

6. General remarks, and perspectives

It has been fascinating to follow the field of mitochondrial diseases research during almost five decades. From my experience, it is impossible to predict which aspects in this area of research will dominate in the future.

Acknowledgements

The author is grateful to his mentors: Rodolfo Brenner and Phillip Strittmatter, all his Ph.D. students, and post docs.

Author details

Angel Catala[1,2]

1 Facultad de Ciencias Exactas, Instituto de Investigaciones Fisicoquímicas Teóricas y Aplicadas (INIFTA-CCT La Plata-CONICET), Universidad Nacional de La Plata, Argentina

2 Consejo Nacional de Investigaciones Científicas y Técnicas (CONICET), Argentina

*Address all correspondence to: catala@inifta.unlp.edu.ar

References

[1] Catala A. (2013) Five Decades with Polyunsaturated Fatty Acids: Chemical Synthesis, Enzymatic Formation, Lipid Peroxidation and Its Biological Effects J Lipids. Available online: https://www.hindawi.com/journals/jl/2013/710290/ [PMC free article]

[2] Catala A. (2009). Lipid peroxidation of membrane phospholipids generates hydroxyl-alkenals and oxidized phospholipids active in physiological and/or pathological conditions. Chem. Phys. Lipids 157, 1-11

[3] Gonzalvez F., Gottlieb E. (200/) Cardiolipin: setting the beat of apoptosis. Apoptosis: An International Journal on Programmed Cell Death. 12:877-885.

[4] Yin H., Zhu M. (2012) Free radical oxidation of cardiolipin: chemical mechanisms, detection and implication in apoptosis, mitochondrial dysfunction and human diseases. Free Radical Research. 46:959-974

Chapter 2

Mitochondria and Eye

Lata Singh and Mithalesh Kumar Singh

Abstract

Mitochondria are essential subcellular organelles and important key regulators of metabolism. Mammalian mitochondria contain their own DNA (mtDNA). Human mtDNA is remarkably small (16,569 bp) compared to nuclear DNA. Mitochondria promote aerobic respiration, an important part of energy metabolism in eukaryotes, as the site of oxidative phosphorylation (OXPHOS). OXPHOS occurs in the inner membrane of the mitochondrion and involves 5 protein complexes that sequentially undergo reduction-oxygen reactions ultimately producing adenosine triphosphate (ATP). Tissues with high metabolic demand such as lungs, central nervous system, peripheral nerves, heart, adrenal glands, renal tubules and the retina are affected preferentially by this critical role in energy production by mitochondrial disorders. Eye-affected mitochondrial disorders are always primary, but the role of mitochondrial dysfunction is now best understood in acquired chronic progressive ocular diseases. Recent advances in mitochondrial research have improved our understanding of ocular disorders. In this chapter, we will discuss the mitochondria in relation to eye diseases, ocular tumors, pathogenesis, and treatment modalities that will help to improve the outcomes of these conditions.

Keywords: mitochondria, LHON, biomarkers, mutations, tumors

1. Introduction

1.1 Mitochondria

Mitochondria are essential sub cellular mammalian organelles found in eukaryotes. It is surrounded by two lipid bilayers which is commonly associated with oxidative phosphorylation, a process that meets the majority of cellular energy demands. It is involved in many other cellular functions such as fatty acids oxidation, apoptosis, heme biosynthesis, metabolism of amino acids and lipids, and signal transduction [1]. They are central organelles controlling the life and death of the cell. Mitochondria contain their own DNA, which is maternally inherited. Mitochondrial density varies from one tissue to another [2]. Mitochondrial diseases are heterogeneous group of disorders, often characterized by morphological changes in the mitochondria, a defective respiratory chain and variable symptoms, ranging from severe metabolic disorders with onset in early infancy or childhood to late onset adult myopathies [3]. Mutations in mitochondrial DNA (mtDNA) are the most frequent cause of mitochondrial diseases in adults. However, the mtDNA encodes only a subset of proteins of the different complexes of the respiratory chain [4]. Nuclear genes encode all the other mitochondrial proteins and most of the mitochondrial disorders are caused by mutations in the nuclear genes [5].

IntechOpen

Mitochondria are ~0.5 to ~3 μm long tubular organelles that undergo continuous remodeling of their network by fusion and fission events [6]. Mitochondria forms an extensive network preserved in many cells by an intricate balance between fission and fusion, mitochondrial biogenesis and mitophagy [7, 8]. Mitochondria was identified as the main source of cell energy, and indeed mitochondria is a major site of ATP and macromolecule development. Equivalent-reducing electrons are fuelled by the ETC to produce an electrochemical gradient required for both the production of ATP and the active transport of selective metabolites, such as pyruvate and ATP, through the IMM [9]. Mitochondria, however, plays a variety of roles beyond energy production, including generation of reactive oxygen species (ROS), redox molecules and metabolites, control of cell signaling and cell death, and biosynthetic metabolism.

While mitochondria is best known for harvesting and storage of energy released by oxidation of organic substrates under aerobic conditions by respiration, their many anabolic functions are often ignored [7]. Biosynthetic functions of mitochondria are essential for tumorigenesis and tumor progression [10]. Tumor cells easily survive under hypoxic conditions by recycling NADH to NAD+ through lactate dehydrogenase (LDH) and plasma membrane electron transport (PMET) to enable continued production of glycolytic ATP [11].

2. Mitochondrial genetics

The human mitochondrial genome consists of 16,569 pairs of nucleotides of double-stranded, closed-circular molecules. It was first sequenced in 1981 and updated in 1999 [12, 13]. mtDNA contains no introns and only encodes 13 polypeptides, 22 transfer RNAs (tRNAs), and the mitochondrial protein synthesis genes 12S and 16S rRNA [14]. The 13 polypeptides of the respiratory complexes (RC) encode subunits (7 of 45 for RC-I, 1 of 11 for RC-III, 3 of 13 for RC-IV, and 2 of 16 for RC-V). Along with the remaining 85% of the other RC subunits, the four subunits that make up RC-II are nuclear-encoded [14]. About 22,000 proteins are encoded by nuclear DNA, about 1,500 of which contribute to the mitochondrial proteome. These nuclear encoded proteins include TCA cycle enzymes, amino acids, nucleic acid and lipid biosynthesis, mtDNA and RNA polymerases, transcription factors, and ribosomal proteins, in addition to all DNA pathway repair components. In the cytoplasm, these proteins are expressed and folded through the TOM/TIM complex upon entry through the mitochondrial outer membrane. From there, they find the outer mitochondrial membrane (OMM), the IMM, the intermembrane space (IMS) or the mitochondrial matrix at their specific positions [15]. There is no structural association of mtDNA with histones, as is nuclear DNA. Rather, it is closely associated with a variety of proteins, about 100 nm in diameter, in discrete nucleoids.

Germline mutations resulting in reduced or lost expression of succinate dehydrogenase (SDH), fumarate hydratase (FH) and isocitrate dehydrogenase have been identified in inherited paragangliomas, gastrointestinal stromal tumors, pheochromocytomas, myomas, SDH, papillary renal cell cancer (FH) and gliomas [16]. mtDNA mutations have been involved in neuromuscular and neurodegenerative mitochondrial disease [17–19] and complex diseases such as diabetes [20], cardiovascular disease [21, 22], gastrointestinal disorders [23], skin disorders [24], aging [25, 26] and cancer. Different human populations have different human mtDNA haplotypes, each with a specific mtDNA polymorphism fingerprint, transmitted through the maternal germline. These haplotypes are associated with the geographic origin of the population. Some human haplotypes are at greater risk of developing a certain form of cancer or neurodegenerative disorder during their lifetime than others [27–29]. The 22 mitochondrial tRNA genes have more than 50 percent of the mtDNA mutations involved in carcinogenesis [29].

The single nucleotide polymorphism, 3243A > G, which alters leucine mt-tRNA and thus affects the translation of 13 respiratory subunits, leading to fewer mitochondrial subunits and impaired OXPHOS, is the most common mtDNA mutation [30, 31]. Individuals can develop maternally inherited diabetes and deafness with 10–30 percent defective copies of tRNALeu. Mitochondrial encephalomyopathy, lactic acidosis, and stroke-like episodes (MELAS) are likely to occur in people with 50–90% defective copies [20, 30–35]. The mutation of tRNALeu results in variable types of mitochondrial RC deficiency in various patients. By far, complex I (RC-I) deficiency is the most common finding in MELAS, although some patients have combined RC-I, RC-III and RC-IV deficiencies [30, 36]. Other mutations in mt-tRNA that play a role in human disease include: tRNAlys, which is associated with myoclonal epilepsy, tRNASer with deafness, and tRNAIle with cardiomyopathy [21].

3. Drivers of mtDNA mutations

mtDNA mutations are caused by ROS-mediated oxidative damage [28, 37]. ROS generation in the respiratory chain is an inherent part of OXPHOS. ROS plays an important role in many signaling processes and their levels are regulated by the antioxidant enzyme systems in the mitochondrial matrix and the IMS. However, in situations where OXPHOS is compromised due to misshapen respiratory complexes resulting in increased leakage of electrons to oxygen, ROS levels can overwhelm the antioxidant protection system and damage to nearby mtDNA [38, 39]. DeBalsi and colleagues suggest that errors produced by mtDNA replication and repair machines may also cause mtDNA mutations [40].

Human cells contain 17 different human DNA polymerases, but in mtDNA replication and repair, only polymerase gamma (Pol-γ) functions. A catalytic subunit and an accessory subunit consist of a nuclear-encoded Pol-γ holo-enzyme [40]. Pol-γ replicates high fidelity mtDNA with one misinsertion in every 500,000 new base pairs due to nucleotide selectivity and proofreading capacity [41]. More than 300 Pol-γ mutations have been associated with human illness, some of which occur in adulthood and are associated with aging, including different types of progressive external ophthalmoplegia (PEO) and Parkinson's disease (PD) [40]. The role of Pol-γ in restricting mtDNA mutations has been demonstrated by homozygous, but not heterozygous, mutator mice with re-reading-deficient Pol-g developing multiple age-related disorders and shortening their lifespan. As their antioxidant capacities were the same and the degree of oxidative damage was comparable to wild-type mice, they acquired mtDNA mutations that were not caused by oxidative damage.

Somatic point mutations, great deletions and several linear deleted mtDNA fragments were acquired by the mutator mice. The mtDNA-specific Twinkle helicase, which unwinds mtDNA for Pol-γ synthesis, is another n-mitoprotein involved in mtDNA replication [42]. Overexpression of Twinkle in transgenic mice resulted in increased copy number of mtDNA and OXPHOS and some twinkle mutations are associated with mitochondrial myopathy [40]. Oxidative damage and defective replication are both likely to add to the overall mutational load of the mtDNA cell, and the contribution of each mutational driver is likely to change over time. Inevitable respiratory electron leakage from complexes I and III results in the formation of superoxide, O_2^- that can react with lipids, proteins and DNA [43–46]. Superoxide can be quickly converted to H_2O_2 either naturally or through a manganese superoxide dismutase (MnSOD) dysmutation reaction, a resident of the mitochondrial matrix. In the presence of redox active metal ions, H_2O_2 can generate a highly reactive hydroxyl radical through the Fenton reaction (OH-) [47]. Multiple mtDNA damage sites, including single and double-strand breaks, abasic sites and base changes, are responsible for the OH-radical. Another oxidative burden is caused by damage to mitochondrial protein centers caused by O_2^- to Fe-S and involves subunits of complexes I, II and III as well as aconitase [48–50]. A significant target for ROS is provided by Labile Fe-S enzymes such as mitochondrial aconitase.

Mitochondria located in cells exposed to visible light generate ROS through interactions with mitochondrial photosensitizers, such as cytochrome c oxidase, of particular relevance to the eye, to produce ROS and mtDNA damage [50, 51]. Transferring energy from photoactivated chromophores to oxygen contributes to the formation of singlet oxygen, $^1O_2$, which occurs in an excited state. $^1O_2$ can produce ROS, such as O_2^- by interacting with diatomic oxygen and directly reacting with dual-bond electrons without the formation of free radical intermediates [52]. It is also important to remember that, from non-mitochondrial sources, various tissues within the eye may also produce substantial amounts of ROS. For instance, lipofuscin (an age-related pigment that accumulates with age in RPE cells) is a potent photo-inducible ROS generator, and NADPH oxidase is considered to be a major source of superoxide in microvascular endothelial cells. Studies indicate that ROS may also contribute to exogenous mitochondrial oxidative damage, exacerbating mitochondrial dysfunction [51, 53, 54].

4. Ophthalmologic mitochondrial dysfunction

Mitochondrial disease can manifest in any organ at any age. In general terms, tissues and organs (retina, optic nerve, brain, heart, testis, muscle, etc.) that are heavily dependent upon oxidative phosphorylation bear the brunt of the pathology. It is also puzzling that many mitochondrial disorders affect multiple organ systems, whereas others have a highly stereotyped and organ specific phenotype. These subtle interactions between nuclear and mitochondrial genes in health and disease will have broader relevance for our understanding of many inherited and sporadic disorders.

Mitochondrial disorder can be categorized according to several different criteria in the manifestations of ophthalmology diseases. They may be defined as isolated or nonisolated, occurring in combination with other manifestations of the organ. The dominant trait of the phenotype or a nondominant attribute can be ophthalmologic manifestations. Mitochondrial disorders with ophthalmic manifestations may be caused either by mutations in mtDNA or nuclear DNA. Ophthalmologic symptoms may be unique to syndromic mitochondrial disorder (e.g. Leber hereditary optic neuropathy) or nonspecific to syndromic mitochondrial disorder (eg, cataract). The cornea, iris, lens, ciliary body, retina, choroid, uvea, or optic nerve may be the primary manifestations of ophthalmologic mitochondrial disorder. There is growing evidence supporting an association between mitochondrial dysfunction and a number of ophthalmic diseases causing defects in OXPHOS and increased production of ROS triggering the activation of cell death pathway.

5. Corneal dystrophy

Some evidence has been given in recent years that the cornea may be involved in mitochondrial disorders. However, systematic studies have not been performed on this matter. Astigmatism, corneal dystrophy, corneal clouding, or corneal endothelial dysfunction are corneal disorders associated with mitochondrial dysfunction [55, 56]. Loss of SLC4A11 gene activity which is localized to the inner mitochondrial membrane of corneal endothelium, induces oxidative stress and cell death, resulting in Congenital Hereditary Endothelial Dystrophy (CHED) with corneal edema and vision loss [57]. Fuchs endothelial corneal dystrophy (FECD) is characterized by progressive and non-regenerative corneal endothelial loss. Variations in mtDNA affect the susceptibility of FECD. Mitochondrial variant A10398G and Haplogroup I were significantly associated with FECD [58]. There are few studies showing the role of mtDNA in the pathogenesis of FECD. Mitophagy activation leads to decrease in Mfn2 gene level and loss of mitochondrial mass in FECD [59]. In a study of 20 patients, keratoconus was related to increased oxidative stress due to mitochondrial respiratory chain complex-I sequence variation [60]. Progressive external ophthalmoplegia secondarily led to persistent conjunctivitis and keratitis in a patient with Kearns-Sayre Syndrome [61]. Corneal clouding has been documented occasionally in Kearns-Sayre syndrome due to structural changes in the endothelium or Descemet membrane [62]. Numerous distended mitochondria were present in the corneal epithelium in a child with Leigh syndrome due to the m.8993 T > G mutation [63]. There are also non-specific corneal alterations in a patient with Neurogastrointestinal mitochondrial encephalomyopathy [64]. Pathogenesis of type 2 granular corneal dystrophy (GCD2) is associated with alteration of mitochondrial features and functions that causes mutated GCD2 keratocytes, particularly in older cells [65].

6. Mitochondrial encephalomyopathy, lactic acidosis, and episodic stroke-like syndrome (MELAS)

Early onset of the disease and higher level of mtDNA heteroplasmy are associated with a worse prognosis in mitochondrial encephalomyopathy, lactic acidosis, and episodic stroke-like syndrome (MELAS). Iris involvement in mitochondrial disorders has been rarely mentioned in MELAS [66]. The m.3243A > G variant is the most common heteroplasmic mtDNA mutation in MELAS and underlies a spectrum of diseases. Patchy iris stroma atrophy has been identified in a patient carrying the m.3243A > G mutation in the tRNA (Lys) gene [66]. MNRR1 (CHCHD2) is a bi-organellar regulator of mitochondrial function, found to be depleted in MELAS and significantly associated with m.3243A > G mutation (heteroplasmic) in the mtDNA at a level of ~50 to 90% [67]. Ability of the peroxisome proliferator-activated receptor γ (PPARγ) activator pioglitazone (PioG), in combination with deoxyribonucleosides (dNs), improves the mitochondrial biogenesis/respiratory functions in MELAS cybrid cells containing >90% of the m.3243A > G mutation that found to be novel therapies to treat this disease [68]. Induced pluripotent stem cells (iPSCs) are appropriate for studying mitochondrial diseases caused by mtDNA mutations in MELAS. Increase of autophagy inpatient-specific iPSCs generated from fibroblasts are associated with mtDNA mutations and OXPHOS defects in patients with MELAS [69]. Studies demonstrated that defective MRM2 gene causes a MELAS-like phenotype which suggests the genetic screening of the MRM2 gene in patients with a m.3243 A > G negative MELAS-like presentation [70]. Mutations caused by mitochondrial complex I deficiencies by alleviating ketone bodies are also associated with MELAS that leads to recurrent cerebral insults resembling strokes [71].

7. Cataract

Cataracts are the most common lenticular defects of mitochondrial disorders. In mitochondrial disorders, cataract is typically of the posterior subcapsular type [66]. Autophagic dysfunction and abnormal oxidative stress are associated with cataract. Cataract may be a phenotypic characteristic of MELAS syndrome, but a patient with nonsyndromic mitochondrial disorder due to mtDNA deletion has also been documented as an initial manifestation [66, 72, 73]. Oxidative stress plays an important role in cataractogenesis [74, 75]. Mitochondria are found in the epithelium and superficial fiber cells of the lens and it is extremely sensitive to ROS. Interestingly, mitochondria have been confirmed as the main source of ROS generation in these cell types [76]. A number of in vitro studies have shown that human lens cells are particularly sensitive to oxidative insults, where antioxidant activity was inversely proportional to the severity of cataracts [77]. Proteins, lipids and DNA oxidation have been found in cataract lenses [78–80]. Under high glucose conditions, fluctuations in autophagy and oxidative stress are found in mouse lens epithelial cells (LECs) that might attenuate high glucose-induced oxidative injury to LECs [81]. Cataract proteins lose sulfhydryl groups, contain oxidized residues, produce aggregates of high molecular weight and become insoluble [75]. In addition, cataract has been shown to be a symptom of a newly identified mitochondrial disorder called autosomal recessive myopathy, caused by growth factor mutations, increased liver regeneration gene, which affects protein levels of mitochondrial intermembrane space region [82].

8. Leigh syndrome

In mitochondrial disorders, involvement of ciliary body has rarely been reported. Leigh's syndrome is the most common pediatric syndrome, characterized by symmetrical brain lesions, hypotonia, motor and respiratory deficits, and premature death are associated with pathways involved in mitochondrial diseases [83]. A case report showed ocular histopathological finding such as thinning of nerve fibers and ganglion cell layers in the nasal aspect of the macula, mild atrophy of the temporal aspect of the optic nerve head, and numerous distended mitochondria, non-pigmented cilla are associated with the m.8993 T > G mutation in the ATPase6 gene of mtDNA in patient with Leigh's syndrome [63]. In addition, ciliary epithelium was also found to be impaired by a long-chain 3-hydroxyacyl-CoA dehydrogenase deficiency [84]. Dysfunction of mitochondrial complex I are also associated with many brain pathologies including Leigh's syndrome. Mitochondrial complex I activity facilitates organismal survival by its regeneration potential of NAD+, while optimal motor regulation involves mitochondrial complex I bioenergetic function in Leigh's syndrome [85].

9. Retinitis pigmentosa

Retinitis pigmentosa is a central characteristic of Kearns-Sayre syndrome and neuropathic ataxia retinitis pigmentosa syndrome [72]. Typical for Kearns-Sayre syndrome is 'salt and pepper' retinitis, with areas of increased and decreased pigmentation, especially in the equatorial fundus [62]. Pigment retinopathy is only an uncommon characteristic of progressive external ophtalmoplegia and can be milder than in Kearns-Sayre syndrome [72, 86]. Only certain patients with MELAS or MERRF syndrome have mild posterior pole pigment retinopathy [72]. Mild pigmentary defects were also observed in 2 of 20 patients with Leber hereditary optic neuropathy due to mutation m.11778G > A [72]. Small pigment retinal defects have been identified in a 4-year-old female with a COX deficiency [87]. In addition, because of the mutation m.8993 T > GG retinitis pigmentosa has been identified in patients with Leigh syndrome [88].

In a sample of 44 Korean Leigh syndrome patients, pigmentary retinopathy was also observed in 22% of Korean patients [89]. In a study of 14 patients with pontocerebellar hypoplasia, 4 patients presented with retinopathy without disclosing information [90]. Occasionally, retinal dystrophy can manifest with photophobia. In a report of 46 mitochondrial disease patients, 4 had photophobia. Two patients had Leigh syndrome, 1 of which had rod-cone dystrophy on electroretinography, 1 had Kearns-Sayre syndrome with regular electroretinography, and 1 had MERRF syndrome with isoelectric electroretinography [91].

10. Diabetic retinopathy

It has been shown that mitochondrial dysfunction plays a significant role in diabetic retinopathy [92, 93]. Hyperglycemia causes retinal mitochondrial damages that plays a central role in the development of diabetic retinopathy. Retinal mitochondria undergo elevated oxidative stress in diabetes, and complex III is one of the key causes of increased O_2^- [94]. Superoxide levels are elevated in in the retina of diabetic rats and in retinal vascular endothelial cells incubated in high-glucose media [95] and the content of hydrogen peroxide is also increased in the retina of diabetic rats [96]. In diabetes, membrane lipid peroxidation and oxidative DNA damage, the effects of ROS-induced injury, are elevated in the retina [97]. Chronic overproduction of ROS in the retina results in aberrant mitochondrial functions in diabetes [92]. Overproduction of superoxide by the mitochondrial electron transport chain caused by hyperglycemia is considered to cause major hyperglycemic damage pathways by inhibiting the action of GAPDH. However, it is not yet fully understood the mechanism by which hyperglycemia induces an increase in mitochondrial ROS, with some suggesting a direct effect and others an indirect function via high-glucose-induced cytokines [98–101].

Elevated levels of O_2^- activate caspase 3 in retinal capillaries contributes to cell death [92]. Upregulation of superoxide dismutase (SOD2) inhibited increased mitochondrial O2-induced diabetes, restored mitochondrial function, and prevented both in vitro and in vivo vascular pathology [94, 102–104]. However, the timing of such therapies is important because animal studies have shown that oxidative stress not only leads to the development of diabetic retinopathy, but also to the resistance of retinopathy to reversal [105]. The resistance to reversal of diabetic retinopathy may be due to the accumulation of weakened mitochondrial molecules and ROS-induced damage that is not readily removed even after the restoration of high glycemic control. However, the accumulation of advanced glycation end products is also involved in metabolic memory [106]. The mtDNA variation has also been associated with resistance to type 1 diabetes. A single nucleotide modification (C5173A) is associated with resistance to type 1 diabetes in the Japanese population, resulting in a leucine-to-methionine amino acid substitution in the mitochondrially encoded NADH dehydrogenase subunit 2 gene [107]. Similarly, in comparison with the diabetes-prone nonobese diabetic mouse strain, orthologous polymorphism (C4738A), resulting in L-to-M substitution, offers resistance against the development of spontaneous diabetes [108]. Gusdon et al., have shown that the replacement of methionine results in a lower level of development of ROS from complex III [109].

The product of mtDNA mutations is also known to result in many syndromic central nervous system diseases. The most common retinal pathology is pigmentary retinopathy, while optic neuropathy is an uncommon finding in these disorders. Neurogenic atrophy and retinitis pigmentosa syndrome results from point mutations in the mtDNA ATPase-6 gene, usually T8993G variation. Patients usually present with retinitis pigmentosa with or without optic neuropathy and may develop dystonia [110]. Several mtDNA point mutations may result from MELAS, although the A3243G mutation in the tRNALeu gene is the most common. Patients with MELAS undergo stroke-like episodes leading to recurrent retrochiasmal vision loss, but sometimes even to pigmentary retinopathy without optic atrophy [111]. Its contribution to the pathogenesis of maternally inherited diabetes and deafness is also evidenced by the spectrum of disease resulting from the A3243G point mutation [112–114]. This is a multisystemic disease characterized by sensorineural deafness, retinal defects and diabetes, generally occurring in the third to fourth decades of life [115]. The second phenotype is a pattern dystrophy, with diffuse granularity and pigment clumping, marked by relative sparing of the fovea, and retinal pigment epithelium within the vascular retinal arcades. However, with a strong prognosis, visual acuity is retained, despite the degree of atrophy [116, 117].

11. Macular degeneration

Age-related macular degeneration is a neurodegenerative late-onset disorder that shares certain characteristics of Alzheimer's disease. In most cases, the build-up of protein plaques, known as drusen, in the central macular area of the retina involves age-related macular degeneration. Both age-related macular degeneration and Alzheimer's disease pathogenesis can be driven by stress stimuli, including oxidative stress, aging, genetic factors and inflammation, including the deposition of protein plaques in the retina or brain [98]. Similarities in these two disorders are also found in the risk factor gene polymorphisms, APOE, associated with age-related macular degeneration [99, 100] and Alzheimer's disease [101, 102]. The APOE gene controls the homeostasis of triglycerides and cholesterol [103], and the loss of function of APOE has been correlated with the deposit of senile plaques, consisting mainly of amyloid beta peptide [104], which is produced in drusen [105, 106] and is also associated with an additional risk factor for age-related macular degeneration, i.e. complement protein [107, 108]. Evidence shows that the APOE genotype can dictate the risk of stress stimuli, including oxidative stress, aging, genetic factors and inflammation, including the deposition of protein plaques in the retina or brain, can drive both age-related macular degeneration and Alzheimer's disease pathogenesis. Alzheimer's disease and other chronic disorders, primarily because of its effect on regulation of oxidative stress [109]. Age-related macular degeneration is split into two main forms, i.e. the "wet" form induced by leakage into the subretinal space from choroidal neovascularization and the more common "dry" form associated with the accumulation of drusen in the macula [75]. In patients with age-related macular degeneration, there is an increased incidence of large-scale mtDNA rearrangements and deletions in blood [76] and retinas [77, 78]. In the non-coding mtDNA control area (d-loop) in retinas with age-related macular degeneration, which has been found in Alzheimer's disease and other conditions of oxidative stress, there are also increased rates of single nucleotide polymorphisms [79]. An increased rate of mtDNA deletions and single nucleotide polymorphisms are likely to decrease the amount and density of mitochondria [80].

Other than pigmentary retinopathy or macular degeneration, retinal anomalies include retinal dystrophy, retinal hypertrophy, and pigmentary maculopathy. Patients with Kearns-Sayre syndrome, Leigh syndrome, MELAS syndrome, MERRF syndrome, and Leber hereditary optic neuropathy will find retinal dystrophies that are most easily measured by electroretinography [91]. Retinal hypertrophy has been identified in patients with autosomal recessive spastic ataxia with leukoencephalopathy and autosomal recessive spastic ataxia with Charlevoix-Saguenay (ARSAL/ARSACS) [118]. Six affected males in a family with Mohr-Tranebjaerg syndrome had blindness resulting from unexplained retinal degeneration [119]. Treatment options for retinopathy are usually limited.

12. Choroidal dystrophy

Choroid and uvea are occasionally affected by mitochondrial disorders. Choroid atrophy is the most common manifestation of mitochondrial disorders [66]. Choroidal atrophy was especially identified in the sense of MELAS syndrome [66]. Choroid pigment epithelium atrophy also occurs in maternally inherited deafness and diabetes [120]. Central choroidal dystrophy was identified in 1 patient with Mohr-Tranebjaerg syndrome as confirmed by electroretinography [119]. In addition, chorioretinal dystrophy was reported in a single patient with a significant deletion of mtDNA [121].

13. Uveitis

A significant causative factor causing blindness from retinal photoreceptor degeneration is intraocular inflammation, also referred to as uveitis. Activated macrophages, which generate various cytotoxic agents, including inducible nitric oxide generated by inducible nitric oxide synthase, O_2^- and other ROS, are responsible for oxidative retinal damage in uveitis [122]. Oxidative stress plays an important role in the early stages of experimental autoimmune uveitis (EAU) in the photoreceptor mitochondria. mtDNA damage has been shown to occur early in the EAU; interestingly, nDNA damage occurred later in the EAU [123]. In addition, peroxynitrite-mediated nitration modifies mitochondrial proteins in the inner segments of the photoreceptor, which, in turn, contributes to increased mitochondrial ROS generation [124]. MnSOD has been shown to be upregulated during EAU to promote an increased state of mitochondrial oxidative stress, possibly to combat ROS [125]. In the early phase of the EAU, before leukocyte infiltration, recent data seem to indicate a causative function of oxidative mtDNA harm. Such mitochondrial oxidative damage can be the initial event that contributes to retinal degeneration in uveitis [123].

14. Optic atrophy

Optic atrophy is the principal mitochondrial dysfunction manifestation of the optic nerve. Optic atrophy is a prevalent manifestation of mitochondrial disorder but is often overlooked or misinterpreted. This is due to the difficulties of optic atrophy diagnosis. Funduscopy can more reliably determine optic atrophy if the distal portion of the optic nerve is impaired, or if the more proximal portions of the nerve are affected by orbital magnetic resonance imaging (MRI). A decreased amplitude of visually evoked potential is a sign of optic nerve atrophy [126]. Optic atrophy has been specifically identified in Leber hereditary optic neuropathy and autosomal dominant optic atrophy among syndromic mitochondrial disorders, conditions in which optic atrophy is the dominant phenotypic function [127]. MELAS syndrome, Kearns-Sayre syndrome, Pearson syndrome, pontocerebellar hypoplasia, Mohr-Tranebjaerg syndrome, Alpers-Huttenlocher disease or Wolfram syndrome have been documented more rarely, with optic atrophy [62, 90, 91, 127]. In patients with MERRF syndrome, partial or complete optic atrophy has also been identified [72, 91, 128]. Optical atrophy is a common phenotypic characteristic of inherited motor and sensory neuropathy type VI (HMSN-IV) due to MFN1 mutations [127]. In addition, C12orf65 (COXPD7) mutations manifest phenotypicly with optical atrophy and Leigh-like phenotype [129]. Optical atrophy associated with neuropathy ataxia retinitis pigmentosa syndrome due to m.8993 T > G mutation in the ATPase6 gene was only seen in a single family [110]. In a study of 44 Korean patients with Leigh Syndrome, 22.5 per cent of optical atrophy was identified [89]. Optical disk alterations have been observed only in a single patient with mitochondrial neurogastrointestinal encephalomyopathy [64]. Optical atrophy can also be a characteristic of childhood-onset spinocerebellar ataxia [130] or mitochondrial depletion syndrome. 39 Non-syndromic mitochondrial optic atrophy disorders is attributed to ACI1 mutation [131], due to ND5 mutation with cataract and retinopathy [132].

15. Glaucoma

Increased intraocular pressure (Glaucoma) is an unusual phenotypic characteristic of mitochondrial disorders. There are two primary types of glaucoma that can be distinguished, open-angle glaucoma and closed-angle glaucoma. In addition, normotensive and hypertensive glaucoma are distinguished. Open-angle glaucoma is seldom observed in patients with Leber inherited optic neuropathy or autosomal dominant optic atrophy. Funduscopic findings can indicate a mixture of abnormalities common for glaucoma retinopathy and an inherited Leber optic neuropathy fundus [133]. In a single patient with mitochondrial neurogastrointestinal encephalomyopathy, glaucomatous changes in the optic disc were observed by visual field assessment and optical coherence tomography [64]. In a study of 14 patients with pontocerebellar hypoplasia, one presented with glaucoma [90]. Normal pressure glaucoma is associated with polymorphism in the OPA1 gene [134].

Glaucoma has also been identified in a family with Wolfram Syndrome. There are signs that ND5 mutations are associated with the development of open-angle glaucoma. Glaucoma in mitochondrial disorders may be eligible for treatment with drugs or surgery [135, 136]. There is evidence in glaucoma that mitochondrial dysfunction can reduce the bioenergetic status of retinal ganglion cells, leading to increased susceptibility to oxidative stress and apoptotic cell death [93, 137]. Light exposure may also be an oxidative risk factor, reducing mitochondrial function and increasing the development of ROS in ganglion cells [138]. A defective mitochondria has been highly implicated in neuronal apoptosis in the experimental models of glaucoma [139, 140]. The mtDNA abnormalities further support the importance of mitochondrial dysfunction-associated stress as a risk factor for glaucoma patients [141].

16. Nystagmus

The central nervous system or vestibular involvement in mitochondrial disorders may cause nystagmus or roving eye movements and are the most common ophthalmological manifestations as a symptom in patients with pediatric mitochondrial disorder [142]. A Gaze-evoked nystagmus identified in a single patient with "Leber hereditary optic neuropathy plus" who not only possessed the "m.11778G > A" mutation in the hereditary Leber hereditary optic neuropathy gene but also the "m.3394 T > C" mutation [143]. Since patients with MELAS may display irregular eye movements on an eye movement cueing task, ultrasound records of eye movement may show abnormally slow saccadic reactions, prolonged saccades, impaired suppression of reflex eye movements, prolonged reaction during antisaccades, square-wave jerks, or impaired chase [144]. Patients have epilepsy due to MELAS may have epileptic nystagmus, disrupted smooth pursuit, or transient eye divergence, none of which are outward signs [145]. In addition, nystagmus was documented in a patient carrying a point mutation in the DGUOK gene who also had retinal blindness. Nystagmus, which is a common symptom of the disease along with retinitis pigmentosa, was also reported in a patient with nonsyndromic mitochondrial disorder due to the m.15995G > A mutation in the tRNA (Pro) gene manifesting as ataxia, deafness, and leukoencephalopathy [146]. Nystagmus was part of the phenotype in a study of 7 Czech patients with autosomal dominant optic atrophy [147]. Nystagmus is also a common characteristic of ARSAL/ARSACS [148]. Nystagmus was observed in 14 percent in a study of 44 Korean patients with Leigh syndrome [88].

17. Strabismus

Strabismus was the most common ophthalmologic abnormality in a study of 44 Korean patients with Leigh syndrome and was present in 41% of patients [89]. Of the strabismus patients, 13 had exotropia and 5 had esotropia [89]. In some patients with X-linked sideroblast anemia with ataxia, strabismus has also been identified [149]. In 25 percent of juvenile mitochondrial disorders, divergent strabismus has been identified as the presenting manifestation [150]. In a study of 14 patients with pontocerebellar hypoplasia, of whom 13 had a CASK mutation, 2 had strabismus. 9 Strabismus was also identified without knowing the underlying mutation in other patients with pontocerebellar hypoplasia [151, 152]. The initial presentation at birth was cataract and strabismus in a child with a significant mtDNA deletion. Later on, he experienced Leigh-like pathologies and episodes of stroke [153]. In certain instances, surgery can have a beneficial effect on strabism.

18. Progressive external ophthalmoplegia

In mitochondrial disorders, affectation of the extraocular muscles results in progressive external ophthalmoplegia. The recurrent ophthalmologic manifestation of mitochondrial disorders is progressive external ophthalmoplegia. It may be complete, resulting in, or partial, walled-in bulbs. Both directions of bulb movements or only some of them can be affected. One eye or both eyes can be affected by it. Single or multiple mtDNA deletions are most often associated with progressive external ophthalmoplegia. Progressive external ophthalmoplegia, Kearns-Sayre syndrome or Pearson syndrome can cause single mtDNA deletions [154]. Multiple deletions of mtDNA may be due to mutations in nuclear genes such as PEO1, POLG1, SLC25A4, RRM2B, POLG2, or OPA1, along with progressive external ophthalmoplegia [154]. In addition, progressive external ophthalmoplegia, especially in the transfer of RNA (eg, tRNA(Lys)) genes, may be due to mtDNA point mutations [154]. Transfer RNA mutations with progressive external ophthalmoplegia are mostly sporadically similar to mtDNA deletions and can only be observed in muscle deletions [155]. The sole manifestation of the m.3243A > G mutation, which often manifests as MELAS syndrome, may be progressive external ophthalmoplegia [156]. In a patient with mitochondrial neurogastrointestinal encephalomyopathy, progressive external ophthalmoplegia was a phenotypic feature [64], Wolfram syndrome [157], Leigh syndrome, autosomal dominant optic atrophy, and mitochondrial recessive ataxia syndrome. In MERRF syndrome, progressive external ophthalmoplegia has also been described [158].

Infantile-onset spinocerebellar ataxia is a Finnish disorder, with some of the 24 cases identified to date developing ophthalmoplegia [130]. Ophthalmoparesis is a hallmark of sensory ataxic neuropathy with ophthalmoparesis syndrome and dysarthria [159]. Sensory ataxic neuropathy with dysarthria and ophthalmoparesis is due to mutations in either the POLG1 or PEO1 gene resulting in multiple mtDNA deletions [159]. Furthermore, ophthalmoparesis can be observed in patients with mitochondrial depletion syndrome [160] or nonsyndromal mitochondrial disorders [161]. In patients with Leber inherited optic neuropathy and progressive external ophthalmoplegia, ultrastructural variations in muscle biopsy from the extraocular muscles clearly differ [162].

19. Eyelid

Ptosis is one of the most common forms of mitochondrial dysfunction. It can occur unilaterally at onset, but during the course of the disease, it usually becomes bilateral. Ptosis can be the sole manifestation, particularly at the onset of the disease, of a mitochondrial disorder or associated with other manifestations. Particularly at the onset of the disease, ptosis can show dynamic alterations, leading to misinterpretation as myasthenia gravis [163]. Ptosis may be discrete, especially at initiation, so that it is missed on clinical review. Progressive external ophthalmoplegia or other ocular symptoms of mitochondrial disease can be associated with ptosis. Ptosis of syndromic as well as nonsyndromic mitochondrial disorders may be a phenotypic manifestation. In particular, ptosis was identified in progressive external ophthalmoplegia, MELAS, MERRF, Kearns-Sayre syndrome, sensory ataxic neuropathy with dysarthria and ophthalmoparesis [164], Pearson syndrome, mitochondrial neurogastrointestinal encephalomyopathy, and autosomal dominant optic atrophy, among the syndromic mitochondrial disorders [91]. Ptosis was present in 16 percent in a group of 44 Korean patients with Leigh syndrome [89]. Ptosis was also present in isolated cases of maternally inherited deafness and diabetes [156], mitochondrial neurogastrointestinal encephalomyopathy [64], or mitochondrial depletion syndrome [160]. Poor lid closure was found in a Persian Jew with mitochondrial myopathy, lactic acidosis, and sideroblastic anemia due to a PUS1 mutation [165].

20. Leber hereditary optic neuropathy

Leber hereditary optic neuropathy is a maternally inherited blindness condition caused by gene mutations encoding the respiratory-chain complex I subunits. Nearly 90 percent of all cases of Leber inherited optic neuropathy contain mutations in 3 genes [128]. The m.3460A > G mutation in the ND1 gene, the m.11778G > A mutation in the ND4 gene and the m.14484 T > C mutation in the ND6 gene are the 3 most common Leber hereditary optic neuropathy mutations (primary Leber hereditary optic neuropathy mutations) [128]. Leber inherited optic neuropathy is clinically characterized as bilateral, painless, subacute vision impairment that occurs during young adult life [134].

Compared with women, Leber hereditary optic neuropathy is 4 to 5 times more common in males. Individuals affected are usually completely asymptomatic until they experience visual blurring in 1 eye affecting the central visual field [134]. On average, 2 to 3 months later, similar signs develop in the other eye. In most cases, visual acuity is greatly diminished or even worse when counting fingers, and visual field examination reveals an expanded central or ceco-central thick scotoma [134]. After the acute process, the optical disks become atrophic. Funduscopic findings characteristic of Leber inherited optic neuropathy include microangiopathy, hyperemic disks, retinal telangiectasis (ectatic capillaries), peripapillary microangiopathy, and tortuosity of vessels (twisted vessels). (twisted vessels). The orbital MRI can display atrophy of the nerve with a compensated widening of the space below the optic sheath. Mutations in mitochondrial ND3, ND4, or ND6 genes can cause hereditary Leber optic neuropathy with dystonia [166].

21. Autosomal dominant optic atrophy

Autosomal dominant optic atrophy is a blindness condition which does not display a gender disparity, unlike Leber inherited optic neuropathy [127]. It is caused by mutations in the nuclearly encoded OPA1 gene [127]. Autosomal dominant optic atrophy can also be due to OPA3 mutations that are associated with cataract [167]. Progressive, painless, bilateral symmetrical vision loss clinically characterizes autosomal dominant optic atrophy [154]. Central, ceco-central, or para-central scotomas, consistent with early involvement of the papillo-macular bundle, are the most common visual field anomalies in autosomal dominant optic atrophy [154]. OPA1 mutations can manifest not only with optic atrophy in some families, but also with progressive external ophthalmoplegia, ptosis, and hypoacusis [168]. Since glaucoma neuropathy, autosomal dominant optic atrophy, and Leber hereditary optic neuropathy often have similar changes in the topographic optic disc, they cannot be discriminated against alone by disc evaluation [169]. There is currently no appropriate treatment available.

22. Retinoblastoma

Retinoblastoma (Rb) is the most common intraocular cancer in children that arise from retinal precursor cells. Electron microscopy revealed numerous morphological and pathological changes in mitochondria of retinoblastoma patients. Cristolysis and degenerated mitochondria were the most frequently observed features in Rb [170]. A study suggested that T16519C, C16223T, A263G and A73G mtDNA D-Loop mutations plays a significant role in the etiology of retinoblastoma. This was the first study to examine the mtDNA D-loop mutation in retinoblastoma and its correlation with various parameters and patient outcome [171]. Their findings imply a strong inhibition of mitochondrial oxidative phosphorylation complexes in these patients. Loss of mitochondrial complex I was found in majority of the cases whereas expression of mitochondrial complex III, IV and V were found in more than 50% of the cases. Expression of mitochondrial complex I was associated with good prognosis and better overall survival [172]. Another consequence of alteration in OXPHOS complexes is an increased production of reactive oxygen species (ROS). NADPH oxidases (NOX4) are a major intracellular source of ROS and it was found to be overexpressed in retinoblastoma [173]. Increased expression of ROS and decreased expression of OXPHOS complexes modulates the apoptotic pathway involved in mitochondria by altering BCl-2 family proteins. Singh et al. showed a differential expression of apoptotic regulatory proteins (Bax, BCl-2, PUMA and p53) where they found increased expression of BCl-2 and PUMA along with loss of Bax and p53, which might contribute to carcinogenesis in Rb [174].

23. Conclusion

Researchers found that these findings are important because they indicate that mtDNA damage can be caused by both spontaneous ROS and by inherited mtDNA mutations. Continued study in this clinically important area would certainly provide a better understanding of how deficiencies/mutations of the mitochondrial genome contribute to the pathogenesis of ocular diseases. The biggest problems with the future of mitochondria are the advancement of therapeutic strategies to target mitochondria and modify its DNA using nucleotide precursors to retain mitochondrial integrity. These therapeutic strategies can potentially be used to block or slow down the effects of mitochondrial disease in future.

Author details

Lata Singh[1*] and Mithalesh Kumar Singh[2]

1 Department of Pediatric, All India Institute of Medical Sciences, New Delhi, India

2 Department of Dermatology, University of Wisconsin, Madison, USA

*Address all correspondence to: lata.aiims@gmail.com

References

[1] Chandel, N.S., *Mitochondria as signaling organelles.* BMC Biol, 2014. **12**: p. 34.

[2] Taylor, R.W. and D.M. Turnbull, *Mitochondrial DNA mutations in human disease.* Nat Rev Genet, 2005. **6**(5): p. 389-402.

[3] Khan, N.A., et al., *Mitochondrial disorders: challenges in diagnosis & treatment.* Indian J Med Res, 2015. **141**(1): p. 13-26.

[4] Ryzhkova, A.I., et al., *Mitochondrial diseases caused by mtDNA mutations: a mini-review.* Ther Clin Risk Manag, 2018. **14**: p. 1933-1942.

[5] Rusecka, J., et al., *Nuclear genes involved in mitochondrial diseases caused by instability of mitochondrial DNA.* J Appl Genet, 2018. **59**(1): p. 43-57.

[6] Chan, D.C., *Mitochondrial fusion and fission in mammals.* Annu Rev Cell Dev Biol, 2006. **22**: p. 79-99.

[7] Chan, D.C., *Fusion and fission: interlinked processes critical for mitochondrial health.* Annu Rev Genet, 2012. **46**: p. 265-87.

[8] Hoitzing, H., I.G. Johnston, and N.S. Jones, *What is the function of mitochondrial networks? A theoretical assessment of hypotheses and proposal for future research.* Bioessays, 2015. **37**(6): p. 687-700.

[9] Kaback, H.R., *Electrochemical ion gradients and active transport.* Ann N Y Acad Sci, 1980. **339**: p. 53-60.

[10] Ahn, C.S. and C.M. Metallo, *Mitochondria as biosynthetic factories for cancer proliferation.* Cancer Metab, 2015. **3**(1): p. 1.

[11] Herst, P.M. and M.V. Berridge, *Plasma membrane electron transport: a new target for cancer drug development.* Curr Mol Med, 2006. **6**(8): p. 895-904.

[12] Anderson, S., et al., *Sequence and organization of the human mitochondrial genome.* Nature, 1981. **290**(5806): p. 457-65.

[13] Andrews, R.M., et al., *Reanalysis and revision of the Cambridge reference sequence for human mitochondrial DNA.* Nat Genet, 1999. **23**(2): p. 147.

[14] Taanman, J.W., *The mitochondrial genome: structure, transcription, translation and replication.* Biochim Biophys Acta, 1999. **1410**(2): p. 103-23.

[15] Hensen, F., et al., *To be or not to be a nucleoid protein: a comparison of mass-spectrometry based approaches in the identification of potential mtDNA-nucleoid associated proteins.* Biochimie, 2014. **100**: p. 219-26.

[16] Nunnari, J. and A. Suomalainen, *Mitochondria: in sickness and in health.* Cell, 2012. **148**(6): p. 1145-59.

[17] Swerdlow, R.H., *The neurodegenerative mitochondriopathies.* J Alzheimers Dis, 2009. **17**(4): p. 737-51.

[18] Hroudová, J., N. Singh, and Z. Fišar, *Mitochondrial dysfunctions in neurodegenerative diseases: relevance to Alzheimer's disease.* Biomed Res Int, 2014. **2014**: p. 175062.

[19] Finsterer, J., *Cognitive dysfunction in mitochondrial disorders.* Acta Neurol Scand, 2012. **126**(1): p. 1-11.

[20] Li, R. and M.X. Guan, *Human mitochondrial leucyl-tRNA synthetase*

corrects mitochondrial dysfunctions due to the tRNALeu(UUR) A3243G mutation, associated with mitochondrial encephalomyopathy, lactic acidosis, and stroke-like symptoms and diabetes. Mol Cell Biol, 2010. **30**(9): p. 2147-54.

[21] Ylikallio, E. and A. Suomalainen, *Mechanisms of mitochondrial diseases.* Ann Med, 2012. **44**(1): p. 41-59.

[22] Finsterer, J. and S. Zarrouk-Mahjoub, *Mitochondrial vasculopathy.* World J Cardiol, 2016. **8**(5): p. 333-9.

[23] Finsterer, J. and M. Frank, *Gastrointestinal manifestations of mitochondrial disorders: a systematic review.* Therap Adv Gastroenterol, 2017. **10**(1): p. 142-154.

[24] Feichtinger, R.G., et al., *Mitochondrial dysfunction: a neglected component of skin diseases.* Exp Dermatol, 2014. **23**(9): p. 607-14.

[25] Larsson, N.G., *Somatic mitochondrial DNA mutations in mammalian aging.* Annu Rev Biochem, 2010. **79**: p. 683-706.

[26] Taylor, S.D., et al., *Targeted enrichment and high-resolution digital profiling of mitochondrial DNA deletions in human brain.* Aging Cell, 2014. **13**(1): p. 29-38.

[27] Wallace, D.C., *Genetics: Mitochondrial DNA in evolution and disease.* Nature, 2016. **535**(7613): p. 498-500.

[28] van Gisbergen, M.W., et al., *How do changes in the mtDNA and mitochondrial dysfunction influence cancer and cancer therapy? Challenges, opportunities and models.* Mutat Res Rev Mutat Res, 2015. **764**: p. 16-30.

[29] Brandon, M.C., et al., *MITOMAP: a human mitochondrial genome database--2004 update.* Nucleic Acids Res, 2005. **33**(Database issue): p. D611-3.

[30] Goto, Y., I. Nonaka, and *S. horai, A mutation in the tRNA(Leu)(UUR) gene associated with the MELAS subgroup of mitochondrial encephalomyopathies.* Nature, 1990. **348**(6302): p. 651-3.

[31] Sasarman, F., H. Antonicka, and E.A. Shoubridge, *The A3243G tRNALeu(UUR) MELAS mutation causes amino acid misincorporation and a combined respiratory chain assembly defect partially suppressed by overexpression of EFTu and EFG2.* Hum Mol Genet, 2008. **17**(23): p. 3697-707.

[32] Picard, M., et al., *Progressive increase in mtDNA 3243A>G heteroplasmy causes abrupt transcriptional reprogramming.* Proc Natl Acad Sci U S A, 2014. **111**(38): p. E4033-42.

[33] Finsterer, J., *Genetic, pathogenetic, and phenotypic implications of the mitochondrial A3243G tRNALeu(UUR) mutation.* Acta Neurol Scand, 2007. **116**(1): p. 1-14.

[34] Goto, Y., et al., *Mitochondrial myopathy, encephalopathy, lactic acidosis, and stroke-like episodes (MELAS): a correlative study of the clinical features and mitochondrial DNA mutation.* Neurology, 1992. **42**(3 Pt 1): p. 545-50.

[35] Hirano, M. and S.G. Pavlakis, *Mitochondrial myopathy, encephalopathy, lactic acidosis, and strokelike episodes (MELAS): current concepts.* J Child Neurol, 1994. **9**(1): p. 4-13.

[36] Chae, J.H., et al., *Clinical features of A3243G mitochondrial tRNA mutation.* Brain Dev, 2004. **26**(7): p. 459-62.

[37] Lane, N., *Mitonuclear match: optimizing fitness and fertility over generations drives ageing within generations.* Bioessays, 2011. **33**(11): p. 860-9.

[38] Holzerová, E. and H. Prokisch, *Mitochondria: Much ado about nothing? How dangerous is reactive oxygen species production?* Int J Biochem Cell Biol, 2015. **63**: p. 16-20.

[39] Chen, Y., et al., *Mitochondrial Redox Signaling and Tumor Progression.* Cancers (Basel), 2016. **8**(4).

[40] DeBalsi, K.L., K.E. Hoff, and W.C. Copeland, *Role of the mitochondrial DNA replication machinery in mitochondrial DNA mutagenesis, aging and age-related diseases.* Ageing Res Rev, 2017. **33**: p. 89-104.

[41] Longley, M.J., et al., *The fidelity of human DNA polymerase gamma with and without exonucleolytic proofreading and the p55 accessory subunit.* J Biol Chem, 2001. **276**(42): p. 38555-62.

[42] Ding, L. and Y. Liu, *Borrowing nuclear DNA helicases to protect mitochondrial DNA.* Int J Mol Sci, 2015. **16**(5): p. 10870-87.

[43] Brand, M.D., et al., *Mitochondrial superoxide: production, biological effects, and activation of uncoupling proteins.* Free Radic Biol Med, 2004. **37**(6): p. 755-67.

[44] Estabrook, R.W., *Observations on the antimycin A inhibition of biological oxidations. II. Electronic analog computer studies.* Biochim Biophys Acta, 1962. **60**: p. 249-58.

[45] Cadenas, E. and K.J. Davies, *Mitochondrial free radical generation, oxidative stress, and aging.* Free Radic Biol Med, 2000. **29**(3-4): p. 222-30.

[46] Turrens, J.F., A. Alexandre, and A.L. Lehninger, *Ubisemiquinone is the electron donor for superoxide formation by complex III of heart mitochondria.* Arch Biochem Biophys, 1985. **237**(2): p. 408-14.

[47] Ashley, N., et al., *Defects in maintenance of mitochondrial DNA are associated with intramitochondrial nucleotide imbalances.* Human molecular genetics, 2007. **16**(12): p. 1400-1411.

[48] Fridovich, I., *Superoxide anion radical (O· 2), superoxide dismutases, and related matters.* Journal of Biological Chemistry, 1997. **272**(30): p. 18515-18517.

[49] Patel, M., et al., *Requirement for superoxide in excitotoxic cell death.* Neuron, 1996. **16**(2): p. 345-355.

[50] Liang, L.P. and M. Patel, *Iron-sulfur enzyme mediated mitochondrial superoxide toxicity in experimental Parkinson's disease.* Journal of neurochemistry, 2004. **90**(5): p. 1076-1084.

[51] Godley, B.F., et al., *Blue light induces mitochondrial DNA damage and free radical production in epithelial cells.* Journal of Biological Chemistry, 2005. **280**(22): p. 21061-21066.

[52] Min, D. and J. Boff, *Chemistry and reaction of singlet oxygen in foods.* Comprehensive reviews in food science and food safety, 2002. **1**(2): p. 58-72.

[53] Newsholme, P., et al., *Diabetes associated cell stress and dysfunction: role of mitochondrial and non-mitochondrial ROS production and activity.* The Journal of physiology, 2007. **583**(1): p. 9-24.

[54] Whiteside, C.I., *Cellular mechanisms and treatment of diabetes vascular complications converge on reactive oxygen species.* Current hypertension reports, 2005. 7(2): p. 148-154.

[55] Lee, J.J., et al., *A mitochondrial DNA deletion presenting with corneal clouding and severe Fanconi syndrome.* Pediatric Nephrology, 2012. **27**(5): p. 869-872.

[56] Kasbekar, S.A., et al., *Corneal endothelial dysfunction in Pearson syndrome.* Ophthalmic genetics, 2013. **34**(1-2): p. 55-57.

[57] Ogando, D.G., et al., *Ammonia sensitive SLC4A11 mitochondrial uncoupling reduces glutamine induced oxidative stress.* Redox Biol, 2019. **26**: p. 101260.

[58] Li, Y.J., et al., *Mitochondrial polymorphism A10398G and Haplogroup I are associated with Fuchs' endothelial corneal dystrophy.* Invest Ophthalmol Vis Sci, 2014. **55**(7): p. 4577-84.

[59] Benischke, A.S., et al., *Activation of mitophagy leads to decline in Mfn2 and loss of mitochondrial mass in Fuchs endothelial corneal dystrophy.* Sci Rep, 2017. **7**(1): p. 6656.

[60] Pathak, D., et al., *Mitochondrial complex 1 gene analysis in keratoconus.* Molecular vision, 2011. **17**: p. 1514.

[61] Schmitz, K., H. Lins, and W. Behrens-Baumann, *Bilateral spontaneous corneal perforation associated with complete external ophthalmoplegia in mitochondrial myopathy (Kearns-Sayre syndrome).* Cornea, 2003. **22**(3): p. 267-270.

[62] Al-Enezi, M., H. Al-Saleh, and M. Nasser, *Mitochondrial disorders with significant ophthalmic manifestations.* Middle East African journal of ophthalmology, 2008. **15**(2): p. 81.

[63] Hayashi, N., M.T. Geraghty, and W.R. Green, *Ocular histopathologic study of a patient with the T 8993-G point mutation in Leigh's syndrome.* Ophthalmology, 2000. **107**(7): p. 1397-1402.

[64] Barboni, P., et al., *Ocular findings in mitochondrial neurogastrointestinal encephalomyopathy: a case report.* Graefe's Archive for Clinical and Experimental Ophthalmology, 2004. **242**(10): p. 878-880.

[65] Kim, T.I., et al., *Altered mitochondrial function in type 2 granular corneal dystrophy.* Am J Pathol, 2011. **179**(2): p. 684-92.

[66] Rummelt, V., et al., *Ocular pathology of MELAS syndrome with mitochondrial DNA nucleotide 3243 point mutation.* Ophthalmology, 1993. **100**(12): p. 1757-1766.

[67] Aras, S., et al., *Mitochondrial Nuclear Retrograde Regulator 1 (MNRR1) rescues the cellular phenotype of MELAS by inducing homeostatic mechanisms.* Proc Natl Acad Sci U S A, 2020. **117**(50): p. 32056-32065.

[68] Burgin, H.J., et al., *Pioglitazone and Deoxyribonucleoside Combination Treatment Increases Mitochondrial Respiratory Capacity in m.3243A>G MELAS Cybrid Cells.* Int J Mol Sci, 2020. **21**(6).

[69] Lin, D.S., et al., *Oxidative Insults and Mitochondrial DNA Mutation Promote Enhanced Autophagy and Mitophagy Compromising Cell Viability in Pluripotent Cell Model of Mitochondrial Disease.* Cells, 2019. **8**(1).

[70] Garone, C., et al., *Defective mitochondrial rRNA methyltransferase MRM2 causes MELAS-like clinical syndrome.* Hum Mol Genet, 2017. **26**(21): p. 4257-4266.

[71] Frey, S., et al., *The addition of ketone bodies alleviates mitochondrial dysfunction by restoring complex I assembly in a MELAS cellular model.* Biochim Biophys Acta Mol Basis Dis, 2017. **1863**(1): p. 284-291.

[72] Isashiki, Y., et al., *Retinal manifestations in mitochondrial diseases*

associated with mitochondrial DNA mutation. Acta Ophthalmol Scand, 1998. **76**(1): p. 6-13.

[73] Bene, J., et al., *Congenital cataract as the first symptom of a neuromuscular disease caused by a novel single large-scale mitochondrial DNA deletion.* Eur J Hum Genet, 2003. **11**(5): p. 375-9.

[74] Brennan, L.A. and M. Kantorow, *Mitochondrial function and redox control in the aging eye: role of MsrA and other repair systems in cataract and macular degenerations.* Exp Eye Res, 2009. **88**(2): p. 195-203.

[75] Lou, M.F., *Redox regulation in the lens.* Prog Retin Eye Res, 2003. **22**(5): p. 657-82.

[76] Huang, L., et al., *Oxidation-induced changes in human lens epithelial cells 2. Mitochondria and the generation of reactive oxygen species.* Free Radic Biol Med, 2006. **41**(6): p. 926-36.

[77] Spector, A., *Oxidative stress-induced cataract: mechanism of action.* Faseb j, 1995. **9**(12): p. 1173-82.

[78] Yao, K., et al., *Protective effect of magnolol against hydrogen peroxide-induced oxidative stress in human lens epithelial cells.* Am J Chin Med, 2009. **37**(4): p. 785-96.

[79] Hightower, K.R., et al., *Ultraviolet irradiation (UVB) interrupts calcium cell signaling in lens epithelial cells.* Photochem Photobiol, 1999. **69**(5): p. 595-8.

[80] Reddan, J.R., et al., *Protection from oxidative insult in glutathione depleted lens epithelial cells.* Exp Eye Res, 1999. **68**(1): p. 117-27.

[81] Liu, X., et al., *Autophagy attenuates high glucose-induced oxidative injury to lens epithelial cells.* Biosci Rep, 2020. **40**(4).

[82] Di Fonzo, A., et al., *The mitochondrial disulfide relay system protein GFER is mutated in autosomal-recessive myopathy with cataract and combined respiratory-chain deficiency.* Am J Hum Genet, 2009. **84**(5): p. 594-604.

[83] Gella, A., et al., *Mitochondrial Proteome of Affected Glutamatergic Neurons in a Mouse Model of Leigh Syndrome.* Front Cell Dev Biol, 2020. **8**: p. 660.

[84] Tyni, T., et al., *Mitochondrial fatty acid beta-oxidation in the human eye and brain: implications for the retinopathy of long-chain 3-hydroxyacyl-CoA dehydrogenase deficiency.* Pediatr Res, 2004. **56**(5): p. 744-50.

[85] McElroy, G.S., et al., *NAD+ Regeneration Rescues Lifespan, but Not Ataxia, in a Mouse Model of Brain Mitochondrial Complex I Dysfunction.* Cell Metab, 2020. **32**(2): p. 301-308.e6.

[86] Pfeffer, G., et al., *Multisystem disorder in late-onset chronic progressive external ophthalmoplegia.* Can J Neurol Sci, 2011. **38**(1): p. 119-23.

[87] Sieverding, L., et al., *[Encephalomyelopathy, cardiomyopathy, cataract and changes in the retinal pigment epithelium resulting from a cytochrome c oxidase deficiency].* Klin Padiatr, 1988. **200**(5): p. 381-7.

[88] Mori, M., et al., *m.8993T>G-Associated Leigh Syndrome with Hypocitrullinemia on Newborn Screening.* JIMD Rep, 2014. **17**: p. 47-51.

[89] Han, J., et al., *Ophthalmological manifestations in patients with Leigh syndrome.* Br J Ophthalmol, 2015. **99**(4): p. 528-35.

[90] Burglen, L., et al., *Spectrum of pontocerebellar hypoplasia in 13 girls and*

boys with CASK mutations: confirmation of a recognizable phenotype and first description of a male mosaic patient. Orphanet journal of rare diseases, 2012. 7(1): p. 18.

[91] Grönlund, M.A., et al., *Ophthalmological findings in children and young adults with genetically verified mitochondrial disease.* Br J Ophthalmol, 2010. **94**(1): p. 121-7.

[92] Kowluru, R.A., *Diabetic retinopathy: mitochondrial dysfunction and retinal capillary cell death.* Antioxid Redox Signal, 2005. 7(11-12): p. 1581-87.

[93] Tezel, G., *Oxidative stress in glaucomatous neurodegeneration: mechanisms and consequences.* Prog Retin Eye Res, 2006. **25**(5): p. 490-513.

[94] Kanwar, M., et al., *Oxidative damage in the retinal mitochondria of diabetic mice: possible protection by superoxide dismutase.* Invest Ophthalmol Vis Sci, 2007. **48**(8): p. 3805-11.

[95] Kowluru, R.A. and S.N. Abbas, *Diabetes-induced mitochondrial dysfunction in the retina.* Invest Ophthalmol Vis Sci, 2003. **44**(12): p. 5327-34.

[96] Ellis, E.A., et al., *Increased H2O2, vascular endothelial growth factor and receptors in the retina of the BBZ/Wor diabetic rat.* Free Radic Biol Med, 2000. **28**(1): p. 91-101.

[97] Kowluru, R.A. and P.S. Chan, *Oxidative stress and diabetic retinopathy.* Exp Diabetes Res, 2007. **2007**: p. 43603.

[98] Lin, Y., et al., *The hyperglycemia-induced inflammatory response in adipocytes: the role of reactive oxygen species.* J Biol Chem, 2005. **280**(6): p. 4617-26.

[99] Santos, D.L., et al., *Diabetes and mitochondrial oxidative stress: a study using heart mitochondria from the diabetic Goto-Kakizaki rat.* Mol Cell Biochem, 2003. **246**(1-2): p. 163-70.

[100] Yorek, M.A., *The role of oxidative stress in diabetic vascular and neural disease.* Free Radic Res, 2003. **37**(5): p. 471-80.

[101] Busik, J.V., S. Mohr, and M.B. Grant, *Hyperglycemia-induced reactive oxygen species toxicity to endothelial cells is dependent on paracrine mediators.* Diabetes, 2008. **57**(7): p. 1952-65.

[102] Nishikawa, T., et al., *Impact of mitochondrial ROS production in the pathogenesis of insulin resistance.* Diabetes Res Clin Pract, 2007. **77 Suppl 1**: p. S161-4.

[103] Kowluru, R.A., L. Atasi, and Y.S. Ho, *Role of mitochondrial superoxide dismutase in the development of diabetic retinopathy.* Invest Ophthalmol Vis Sci, 2006. **47**(4): p. 1594-9.

[104] Kowluru, R.A., et al., *Overexpression of mitochondrial superoxide dismutase in mice protects the retina from diabetes-induced oxidative stress.* Free Radic Biol Med, 2006. **41**(8): p. 1191-6.

[105] Kowluru, R.A., *Effect of reinstitution of good glycemic control on retinal oxidative stress and nitrative stress in diabetic rats.* Diabetes, 2003. **52**(3): p. 818-23.

[106] Stitt, A.W. and T.M. Curtis, *Advanced glycation and retinal pathology during diabetes.* Pharmacol Rep, 2005. **57 Suppl**: p. 156-68.

[107] Uchigata, Y., et al., *A mitochondrial genotype associated with the development of autoimmune-related type 1 diabetes.* Diabetes Care, 2002. **25**(11): p. 2106.

[108] Mathews, C.E., et al., *mt-Nd2 Allele of the ALR/Lt mouse confers resistance against both chemically induced and autoimmune diabetes.* Diabetologia, 2005. **48**(2): p. 261-7.

[109] Gusdon, A.M., T.V. Votyakova, and C.E. Mathews, *mt-Nd2a suppresses reactive oxygen species production by mitochondrial complexes I and III.* J Biol Chem, 2008. **283**(16): p. 10690-7.

[110] Mäkelä-Bengs, P., et al., *Correlation between the clinical symptoms and the proportion of mitochondrial DNA carrying the 8993 point mutation in the NARP syndrome.* Pediatr Res, 1995. **37**(5): p. 634-9.

[111] Sue, C.M., et al., *Pigmentary retinopathy associated with the mitochondrial DNA 3243 point mutation.* Neurology, 1997. **49**(4): p. 1013-7.

[112] van den Ouweland, J.M., et al., *Mutation in mitochondrial tRNA(Leu)(UUR) gene in a large pedigree with maternally transmitted type II diabetes mellitus and deafness.* Nat Genet, 1992. **1**(5): p. 368-71.

[113] Reardon, W., et al., *Diabetes mellitus associated with a pathogenic point mutation in mitochondrial DNA.* Lancet, 1992. **340**(8832): p. 1376-9.

[114] Michaelides, M., et al., *Macular dystrophy associated with the A3243G mitochondrial DNA mutation. Distinct retinal and associated features, disease variability, and characterization of asymptomatic family members.* Arch Ophthalmol, 2008. **126**(3): p. 320-8.

[115] Rath, P.P., et al., *Characterisation of the macular dystrophy in patients with the A3243G mitochondrial DNA point mutation with fundus autofluorescence.* Br J Ophthalmol, 2008. **92**(5): p. 623-9.

[116] Massin, P., et al., *Prevalence of macular pattern dystrophy in maternally inherited diabetes and deafness. GEDIAM Group.* Ophthalmology, 1999. **106**(9): p. 1821-7.

[117] Van Bergen, N.J., et al., *Mitochondrial disorders and the eye.* Eye Brain, 2011. **3**: p. 29-47.

[118] Ponjavic, V., et al., *Full-field electroretinograms in a family with Mohr-Tranebjaerg syndrome.* Acta Ophthalmol Scand, 1996. **74**(6): p. 632-5.

[119] Dhalla, M.S., U.R. Desai, and D.S. Zuckerbrod, *Pigmentary maculopathy in a patient with Wolfram syndrome.* Can J Ophthalmol, 2006. **41**(1): p. 38-40.

[120] Guillausseau, P.-J., et al., *Maternally inherited diabetes and deafness: a multicenter study.* Annals of internal medicine, 2001. **134**(9_Part_1): p. 721-728.

[121] Barrientos, A., et al., *Sporadic heteroplasmic single 5.5 kb mitochondrial DNA deletion associated with cerebellar ataxia, hypogonadotropic hypogonadism, choroidal dystrophy, and mitochondrial respiratory chain complex I deficiency.* Human Mutation, 1997. **10**(3): p. 212-216.

[122] Bosch-Morell, F., et al., *Role of oxygen and nitrogen species in experimental uveitis: anti-inflammatory activity of the synthetic antioxidant ebselen.* Free Radical Biology and Medicine, 2002. **33**(5): p. 669-675.

[123] Khurana, R.N., et al., *Mitochondrial oxidative DNA damage in experimental autoimmune uveitis.* Investigative ophthalmology & visual science, 2008. **49**(8): p. 3299-3304.

[124] Rajendram, R., S. Saraswathy, and N.A. Rao, *Photoreceptor mitochondrial oxidative stress in early experimental*

autoimmune uveoretinitis. British journal of ophthalmology, 2007. **91**(4): p. 531-537.

[125] Saraswathy, S. and N.A. Rao, *Mitochondrial proteomics in experimental autoimmune uveitis oxidative stress.* Investigative ophthalmology & visual science, 2009. **50**(12): p. 5559-5566.

[126] Heiduschka, P., et al., *Electrophysiological and histologic assessment of retinal ganglion cell fate in a mouse model for OPA1-associated autosomal dominant optic atrophy.* Investigative Ophthalmology & Visual Science, 2010. **51**(3): p. 1424-1431.

[127] Carelli, V., et al., *Retinal ganglion cell neurodegeneration in mitochondrial inherited disorders.* Biochimica et Biophysica Acta (BBA)-Bioenergetics, 2009. **1787**(5): p. 518-528.

[128] La Morgia, C., et al., *Association of the mtDNA m. 4171C> A/MT-ND1 mutation with both optic neuropathy and bilateral brainstem lesions.* BMC neurology, 2014. **14**(1): p. 116.

[129] Heidary, G., et al., *Optic atrophy and a Leigh-like syndrome due to mutations in the c12orf65 gene: report of a novel mutation and review of the literature.* Journal of Neuro-ophthalmology, 2014. **34**(1): p. 39-43.

[130] Lönnqvist, T., *Infantile-onset spinocerebellar ataxia*, in *GeneReviews®[Internet]*. 2018, University of Washington, Seattle.

[131] Metodiev, M.D., et al., *Mutations in the tricarboxylic acid cycle enzyme, aconitase 2, cause either isolated or syndromic optic neuropathy with encephalopathy and cerebellar atrophy.* Journal of medical genetics, 2014. **51**(12): p. 834-838.

[132] Valentino, M., et al., *The 13042G→ A/ND5 mutation in mtDNA is pathogenic and can be associated also with a prevalent ocular phenotype.* Journal of medical genetics, 2006. **43**(7): p. e38-e38.

[133] Inagaki, Y., et al., *Mitochondrial DNA mutations with Leber's hereditary optic neuropathy in Japanese patients with open-angle glaucoma.* Japanese journal of ophthalmology, 2006. **50**(2): p. 128-134.

[134] Yu-Wai-Man, P., et al., *OPA1 increases the risk of normal but not high tension glaucoma.* Journal of medical genetics, 2010. **47**(2): p. 120-125.

[135] Bekir, N.A., K. Güngör, and Ş. Güran, *A DIDMOAD syndrome family with juvenile glaucoma and myopia findings.* Acta ophthalmologica scandinavica, 2000. **78**(4): p. 480-482.

[136] Banerjee, D., et al., *Mitochondrial genome analysis of primary open angle glaucoma patients.* PLoS One, 2013. **8**(8): p. e70760.

[137] Osborne, N., et al., *A hypothesis to suggest that light is a risk factor in glaucoma and the mitochondrial optic neuropathies.* British journal of ophthalmology, 2006. **90**(2): p. 237-241.

[138] Lascaratos, G., et al., *Visible light affects mitochondrial function and induces neuronal death in retinal cell cultures.* Vision research, 2007. **47**(9): p. 1191-1201.

[139] Tatton, W.G., et al., *Maintaining mitochondrial membrane impermeability: an opportunity for new therapy in glaucoma?* Survey of Ophthalmology, 2001. **45**: p. S277-S283.

[140] Mittag, T.W., et al., *Retinal damage after 3 to 4 months of elevated intraocular pressure in a rat glaucoma model.* Investigative ophthalmology & visual science, 2000. **41**(11): p. 3451-3459.

[141] Abu-Amero, K.K., J. Morales, and T.M. Bosley, *Mitochondrial abnormalities in patients with primary open-angle glaucoma.* Investigative ophthalmology & visual science, 2006. **47**(6): p. 2533-2541.

[142] Rose, L.V., et al., *Ophthalmologic presentation of oxidative phosphorylation diseases of childhood.* Pediatr Neurol, 2008. **38**(6): p. 395-7.

[143] Nakaso, K., et al., *Leber's Hereditary Optic Neuropathy with Olivocerebellar Degeneration due to G11778A and T3394C Mutations in the Mitochondrial DNA.* J Clin Neurol, 2012. **8**(3): p. 230-4.

[144] Shinmei, Y., et al., *Ocular motor disorders in mitochondrial encephalopathy with lactic acid and stroke-like episodes with the 3271 (T-C) point mutation in mitochondrial DNA.* J Neuroophthalmol, 2007. **27**(1): p. 22-8.

[145] Choi, S.Y., et al., *Pursuit-paretic and epileptic nystagmus in MELAS.* J Neuroophthalmol, 2012. **32**(2): p. 135-8.

[146] Da Pozzo, P., et al., *A novel mutation in the mitochondrial tRNA(Pro) gene associated with late-onset ataxia, retinitis pigmentosa, deafness, leukoencephalopathy and complex I deficiency.* Eur J Hum Genet, 2009. **17**(8): p. 1092-6.

[147] Liskova, P., et al., *Novel OPA1 missense mutation in a family with optic atrophy and severe widespread neurological disorder.* Acta Ophthalmol, 2013. **91**(3): p. e225-31.

[148] Anesi, L., et al., *Two novel homozygous SACS mutations in unrelated patients including the first reported case of paternal UPD as an etiologic cause of ARSACS.* J Mol Neurosci, 2011. **43**(3): p. 346-9.

[149] Bekri, S., M. D'Hooghe, and P. Vermeersch, *X-Linked Sideroblastic Anemia and Ataxia – RETIRED CHAPTER, FOR HISTORICAL REFERENCE ONLY*, in *GeneReviews(®)*, M.P. Adam, et al., Editors. 1993, University of Washington, Seattle Copyright © 1993-2020, University of Washington, Seattle. GeneReviews is a registered trademark of the University of Washington, Seattle. All rights reserved.: Seattle (WA).

[150] Liu, Z., et al., *A novel Twinkle (PEO1) gene mutation in a Chinese family with adPEO.* Mol Vis, 2008. **14**: p. 1995-2001.

[151] Terman, A. and U.T. Brunk, *Oxidative stress, accumulation of biological 'garbage', and aging.* Antioxid Redox Signal, 2006. **8**(1-2): p. 197-204.

[152] Beckman, K.B. and B.N. Ames, *The free radical theory of aging matures.* Physiol Rev, 1998. **78**(2): p. 547-81.

[153] Harman, D., *Aging: a theory based on free radical and radiation chemistry.* J Gerontol, 1956. **11**(3): p. 298-300.

[154] Gorman, G.S. and R.W. Taylor, *Mitochondrial DNA abnormalities in ophthalmological disease.* Saudi J Ophthalmol, 2011. **25**(4): p. 395-404.

[155] Chinnery, P.F., et al., *A novel mitochondrial tRNA isoleucine gene mutation causing chronic progressive external ophthalmoplegia.* Neurology, 1997. **49**(4): p. 1166-8.

[156] Robberecht, K., et al., *Ptosis as an associated finding in maternally inherited diabetes and deafness.* Ophthalmic Genet, 2010. **31**(4): p. 240-3.

[157] Grosse Aldenhövel, H.B., U. Gallenkamp, and C.A. Sulemana, *Juvenile onset diabetes mellitus, central diabetes insipidus and optic atrophy (Wolfram syndrome)--neurological findings and prognostic implications.* Neuropediatrics, 1991. **22**(2): p. 103-6.

[158] Fukuhara, N., et al., *Myoclonus epilepsy associated with ragged-red fibres (mitochondrial abnormalities): disease entity or a syndrome? Light-and electron-microscopic studies of two cases and review of literature.* J Neurol Sci, 1980. **47**(1): p. 117-33.

[159] Hanisch, F., et al., *SANDO syndrome in a cohort of 107 patients with CPEO and mitochondrial DNA deletions.* J Neurol Neurosurg Psychiatry, 2015. **86**(6): p. 630-4.

[160] Finsterer, J. and U. Ahting, *Mitochondrial depletion syndromes in children and adults.* Can J Neurol Sci, 2013. **40**(5): p. 635-44.

[161] Delgado-Alvarado, M., et al., *Parkinsonism, cognitive deficit and behavioural disturbance caused by a novel mutation in the polymerase gamma gene.* J Neurol Sci, 2015. **350**(1-2): p. 93-7.

[162] Carta, A., et al., *Human extraocular muscles in mitochondrial diseases: comparing chronic progressive external ophthalmoplegia with Leber's hereditary optic neuropathy.* Br J Ophthalmol, 2005. **89**(7): p. 825-7.

[163] Finsterer, J., *Mitochondrial disorder mimicking ocular myasthenia.* Acta Neurol Belg, 2010. **110**(1): p. 110-2.

[164] Tanaka, K., et al., *[A case of sensory ataxic neuropathy, dysarthria, and ophthalmoparesis with multiple mitochondrial DNA deletions].* Rinsho Shinkeigaku, 2013. **53**(3): p. 205-11.

[165] Zeharia, A., et al., *Mitochondrial myopathy, sideroblastic anemia, and lactic acidosis: an autosomal recessive syndrome in Persian Jews caused by a mutation in the PUS1 gene.* J Child Neurol, 2005. **20**(5): p. 449-52.

[166] Wang, K., et al., *Mitochondrial ND3 as the novel causative gene for Leber hereditary optic neuropathy and dystonia.* Neurogenetics, 2009. **10**(4): p. 337-45.

[167] Grau, T., et al., *A novel heterozygous OPA3 mutation located in the mitochondrial target sequence results in altered steady-state levels and fragmented mitochondrial network.* J Med Genet, 2013. **50**(12): p. 848-58.

[168] Payne, M., et al., *Dominant optic atrophy, sensorineural hearing loss, ptosis, and ophthalmoplegia: a syndrome caused by a missense mutation in OPA1.* Am J Ophthalmol, 2004. **138**(5): p. 749-55.

[169] O'Neill, E.C., et al., *Optic disc evaluation in optic neuropathies: the optic disc assessment project.* Ophthalmology, 2011. **118**(5): p. 964-70.

[170] Singh, L., T.C. Nag, and S. Kashyap, *Ultrastructural changes of mitochondria in human retinoblastoma: correlation with tumor differentiation and invasiveness.* Tumour Biol, 2016. **37**(5): p. 5797-803.

[171] Singh, L., et al., *Mutational Analysis of the Mitochondrial DNA Displacement-Loop Region in Human Retinoblastoma with Patient Outcome.* Pathol Oncol Res, 2019. **25**(2): p. 503-512.

[172] Singh, L., et al., *Prognostic significance of mitochondrial oxidative phosphorylation complexes: Therapeutic target in the treatment of retinoblastoma.* Mitochondrion, 2015. **23**: p. 55-63.

[173] Singh, L., et al., *Prognostic significance of NADPH oxidase-4 as an indicator of reactive oxygen species stress in human retinoblastoma.* Int J Clin Oncol, 2016. **21**(4): p. 651-657.

[174] Singh, L., et al., *Expression of pro-apoptotic Bax and anti-apoptotic Bcl-2 proteins in human retinoblastoma.* Clin Exp Ophthalmol, 2015. **43**(3): p. 259-67.

Chapter 3

Mitochondrial Cytopathies of the Renal System

Lovelesh K. Nigam, Aruna V. Vanikar,
Rashmi Dalsukhbhai Patel, Kamal V. Kanodia,
Kamlesh Suthar and Umang Thakkar

Abstract

Mitochondria are major intracellular organelles with a variety of critical roles like adenosine triphosphate production, metabolic modulation, generation of reactive oxygen species, maintenance of intracellular calcium homeostasis, and the regulation of apoptosis. Mitochondria often undergo transformation in both physiological and pathological conditions. New concepts point that mitochondrial shape and structure are intimately linked with their function in the kidneys and diseases related to mitochondrial dysfunction have been identified. Diseases associated with mitochondrial dysfunction are termed as "mitochondrial cytopathies". Evidence support that there is a role of mitochondrial dysfunction in the pathogenesis of two common pathways of end-stage kidney disease, namely, chronic kidney disease (CKD) and acute kidney injury (AKI). Mitochondrial cytopathies in kidneys mainly manifest as focal segmental glomerular sclerosis, tubular defects, and as cystic kidney diseases. The defects implicated are mutations in mtDNA and nDNA. The proximal tubular cells are relatively vulnerable to oxidative stress and are therefore apt to suffer from respiratory chain defects and manifest as either loss of electrolyte or low-molecular-weight proteins. Patients with mitochondrial tubulopathy are usually accompanied by myoclonic epilepsy and ragged red muscle fibers (MERRF), and Pearson's, Kearns-Sayre, and Leigh syndromes. The majority of genetic mutations detected in these diseases are fragment deletions of mtDNA. Studies have shown significantly increased ROS production, upregulation of COX I and IV expressions, and inactivation of complex IV in peripheral blood mononuclear cells of patients with stage IV–V CKD, thereby demonstrating the close association between mitochondrial dysfunction and progression to CKD. Furthermore, the mechanisms that translate cellular cues and demands into mitochondrial remodeling and cellular damage, including the role of microRNAs and lncRNAs, are examined with the final goal of identifying mitochondrial targets to improve treatment of patients with chronic kidney diseases.

Keywords: mitochondrial cytopathies, renal, glomerular, mitophagy, fission, fusion

1. Introduction

Mitochondria, also called as the "power house" of the cell, are double membraned cell organelles involved with converting the energy derived from oxidative phosphorylation into a "fuel" in the form of adenosine triphosphate (ATP) [1, 2]. These also are involved in calcium storage, regulation of metabolism and apoptosis, and cell signaling. The energy demand of an organ is directly proportional to the number of mitochondria present in the organ, so heart is the organ with maximum number of mitochondria followed by kidneys [3, 4]. In the kidneys, renal tubular cells are richest in mitochondria, so as to facilitate the energy-consuming task of reabsorption of the majority of the glomerular filtrate. The renal function depends on interplay between multiple cell types, including endothelial cells, podocytes, mesangial cells, and tubulointerstitial cells, and is energetically demanding and relying on mitochondrial function [5].

Renal dysfunction is a multifactorial entity and manifests as a sequel to an acute or chronic insult to the organ. Recently it has been proposed that renal inflammation and tissue damage during acute kidney injury (AKI) and chronic kidney disease (CKD) have been linked to mitochondrial structural and functional alterations [4, 6].

2. Definition

Diseases related to mitochondrial alterations are known as 'mitochondrial cytopathies' (MC) and encompass a group of disorders characterized by mutations either in mitochondrial DNA (mtDNA) or nuclear DNA (nDNA) genes that encode for mitochondrial proteins [6]. Mitochondrial cytopathies affecting the kidneys are broadly classified as [6, 7]:

1. Inherited mitochondrial cytopathies
2. Acquired mitochondrial cytopathies

Mitochondrial cytopathies can also present as:

1. Tubular defects affecting the:
    a. Proximal tubules
    b. Distal tubules.
2. Non-tubular include:
    a. Glomerular diseases
    b. Tubulointerstitial nephritis
    c. Renal cystic diseases
    d. Neoplasia

3. Mechanism of mitochondrial cytopathies

Various studies indicate that mitochondrial dysfunction can arises due to disturbances in the regulation of the mitochondrial electron transport chain, proton gradient, and membrane potential [4, 7]. These disturbances lead to reduction in concentration of adenosine triphosphate (ATP) and increase in production of mitochondrial-derived reactive oxygen species (mROS). These reactive oxygen species promote kidney injury and inflammation [4, 7, 8].

Structural changes of mitochondrial swelling and fragmentation occur earlier than rise in serum creatinine which is largely used as a marker for kidney injury. These changes also indicate that impaired mitochondrial metabolism is directly linked to the deterioration of kidney function [4–9].

Inherited forms of mitochondrial cytopathies are associated with fair number of mutations with mitochondrial DNA (mtDNA) as many nuclear genes are responsible for proper maintenance of mtDNA. Mutations in these genes cause quantitative (mtDNA depletion) and qualitative defects (mtDNA deletions) in mtDNA leading to renal impairment [10].

The equilibrium between mitochondrial fusion and fission maintains the healthy mitochondrial structure and functions [4, 11]. Disruption of this balance leads to mitochondrial fragmentation, loss of mitochondrial DNA (mtDNA) integrity, and cell death [12, 13].

Mitochondrial cytopathies encompasses a group of disorders characterized by mitochondrial or nuclear DNA mutations in genes encoding for mitochondrial proteins [7]. Mitochondrial dysfunction, characterized by a loss of efficiency in the electron transport chain and reductions in the synthesis of high-energy molecules, such as adenosine-5′-triphosphate (ATP), is characteristic of aging, and essentially, of all chronic diseases [1–4]. Mitochondrial dysfunction arises from an inadequate number of mitochondria, an inability to provide necessary substrates to mitochondria, or a dysfunction in their electron transport and ATP-synthesis machinery [10, 11].

The number and functional status of mitochondria in a cell can be changed by [10, 12, 14].

1. Fusion of partially dysfunctional mitochondria and mixing of their undamaged components to improve overall function,

2. The generation of entirely new mitochondria (fission), and.

3. The removal and complete degradation of dysfunctional mitochondria (mitophagy).

3.1 Fission and fusion

The mitochondrial homeostasis is maintained because of the balance between fission and fusion. Fission leads to production of short rods or spheres whereas fusion leads to production of long and filamentous mitochondria. The balance between the two processes is disrupted under stress that leads to mitochondrial fragmentation. The both two processes are mediated by following factors: [15–19]

1. Fission: Fis1(Fission protein 1), Drp1 (Drosophilia 1), Bif-1.

2. Fusion: Mfn 1 and Mfn 2 (Mitochondrial fusion protein 1 & 2), Optic atrophy factor 1 (OPA1).

3.2 The process of fission

Fission is regulated by two main mediators: Drp1 and Fis1. The Drp1 is a GTPase of dynamin superfamily and is mainly present in the cytoplasm and later localizes to the outer membrane of the mitochondria. It has been seen that this shuffling of Drp1 is regulated by phosphorylation, ubiquilation and sumoylation.

Fis1 is a small membrane protein anchored at the outer mitochondrial membrane and overexpression of Fis1 promoted mitochondrial fission causes fragmentation of the mitochondria.

3.3 The process of fusion

Mitochondrial fusion is mediated by mitofusin 1 (Mfn1), mitofusin 2 (Mfn2) and optic atrophy factor 1 (OPA1). All three proteins are GTPases belonging to dynamin superfamily like Drp1. Mfn1 and Mfn2 are also localized to outer mitochondrial membrane whereas OPA1 is present on the inner mitochondrial membrane.

3.4 Mitophagy

Mitophagy, an autophagy process by which dysfunctional or superfluous mitochondria are selectively eliminated. Defective mitophagy has been implicated in various human diseases, such as aging, neurodegenerative disease, cardiovascular disease, cancers and many other renal diseases. Altered mitophagy related mechanisms are implicated in the pathogenesis of acute kidney injury, diabetic kidney disease, and lupus nephritis. The process includes initiation, priming of mitochondria for recognition by autophagy machinery, formation of the autophagosome, followed by lysosomal sequestration and hydrolytic degradation [17–19].

Mitophagy as described by Palikaras, can be described as three types: basal, programmed and stress-induced. Basal mitophagy is a steady-state, continuous, process responsible for elimination and recycling of aged and damaged mitochondria. This type of mitophagy exhibits tissue-specific distribution, with low levels in the thymus and high levels in the heart and kidneys [20, 21]. Stress induced mitophagy facilitates mitochondrial quality control to mediate metabolic adjustments to external challenges [20, 21].

Mitophagy is largely explained by molecular pathways and is mediated by either PINK1/Parkin-pathway or via the receptors. Mitophagy receptors are localized in the outer and inner mitochondrial membranes, and can directly induce mitophagy. Proteins that promote mitophagy are FUN14 domain-containing protein 1, BNIP3 and BCL2 interacting protein 3 like, and FKBP prolyl isomerase 8 [22–24].

Recently it was described that BNIP3/NIX, atypical members of the pro-apoptotic BCL2 family, contain an atypical BH3 domain which under hypoxic stress, get upregulated by hypoxia-inducible factor 1 (HIF-1). This in turn causes initiation of LC3-dependent mitophagy and overproduction of mtROS overproduction [4, 6, 9, 20, 23].

Overall, it is believed that impairment of mitophagy is responsible for mitochondrial dysfunction and progressive accumulation of defective organelles, leading to cell death and tissue damage. Blockade of mitophagy leads to the accumulation of damaged, ROS-generating mitochondria which activate the NLRP3 inflammasome [25].

Thus, mitochondrial cytopathies result due to disturbances in the process related to mitophagy or due to imbalance between the processes of fusion and fission.

4. Mitochondrial dysfunction and kidney injury

In this section we will discuss about the diseases that affect the kidney due to mitochondrial dysfunction. As described before renal mitochondrial cytopathies can manifests either as glomerular or tubular diseases, or as renal cysts or neoplasia.

4.1 Glomerular involvement in renal mitochondrial cytopathies

4.1.1 Diabetic nephropathy

Diabetic nephropathy results from microvascular complications, leading to chronic kidney disease that develops in approximately 30% of patients with type 1 diabetes mellitus (DM1) and approximately 40% of patients with type 2 diabetes mellitus (DM2) [26–28]. Various mitochondrial defects seen include impaired respiratory chain functions, structural and networking abnormalities, disrupted cellular signaling and increased reactive oxygen species generation [4, 29].

Coughlan et al. demonstrated that a deficiency in apoptosis inducing factor (AIF) results in changes in mitochondrial function, networking, and production of reactive oxygen species that precipitate renal disease. Along with the diabetic milieu, switch from mitochondrial fusion to fission, impaired OXPHOS, and a depleted mitochondrial ATP pool, all accelerate towards a more advanced renal injury [30].

Studies have implicated impaired mitophagy as the cause of mitochondrial dysfunction in diabetic kidneys and also showed that with progression of disease, concomitant accumulation of fragmented and swollen mitochondria occurs [22, 30, 31].

Experimental studies have shown that there is decrease in PINK1 and Parkin in the tubules of diabetic mice [32]. In study on streptozotocin-induced diabetic rat models, the authors demonstrated that in early stages of diabetes there is increase in expression of PINK1 in the renal cortex. This provided an evidence that mitophagy could be activated to clear dysfunctional mitochondria from the kidney during early diabetes and as the disease progresses there is accumulation of fragmented mitochondria and induction of cell death [4]. Thioredoxin-interacting protein (TXNIP) - dependent activation of the mammalian target of rapamycin (mTOR) signaling pathway contributes to dysfunctional mitophagy in the diabetic kidney [4, 30, 33, 34].

Studies have evaluated presence of cell-free mtDNA in urine in patients of diabetic nephropathy and reported an inverse relationship in levels of urinary mtDNA and intra-renal mtDNA leading to increase in interstitial fibrosis and reduction in estimated glomerular filtration rate (eGFR) [35].

It has also been demonstrated that damaged mitochondria generate excess mitochondrial superoxide, and glycation of mitochondrial proteins also contributes to mROS generation. Advanced glycation end products as well as the receptors for these, play a vital role in generation of ROS that contribute in progression of diabetic nephropathy [33, 36].

4.1.2 IgA nephropathy (IgAN)

IgAN is one of the most common glomerulonephritis and a leading cause of CKD that can progress to ESRD. Kidney biopsy from a patient with IgAN may show varied morphological affection ranging from mesangial proliferation to focal segmental mesangial sclerosis, crescents with dominant mesangial IgA deposition [4, 37]. The disease is characterized by presence of circulating and glomerular immune complexes comprised of galactose-deficient IgA1, an IgG autoantibody directed against the hinge region O-glycans, and C3 [38]. Nishida et al. demonstrated an increased number of abnormal mitochondria in the proximal tubular epithelial cells and an elevated urinary mtDNA levels in patients with IgAN. An association between five common single-nucleotide polymorphisms and ESRD, suggests that mitochondrial defects have an essential role in the progression to CKD in patients with IgAN [4, 39]. Interestingly, higher expression and interaction between the mitochondrial protein induced in high glucose-1 (IHG-1) and cold shock protein Y-box binding protein-1 are associated with renal inflammation, tubulointerstitial inflammation, and glomerulosclerosis in IgAN. Defects in the mitochondrial genome and functions play a critical role in worsening glomerular inflammation and disease progression [40].

4.1.3 Polycystic kidney disease

Autosomal dominant PKD (ADPKD), is characterized by presence of multiple cysts in the renal parenchyma and is associated with mutations in the genes PKD1 and PKD2, which encode polycystin 1 (PC1) and PC2, respectively [41]. The PC1-PC2 complex modulates mitochondrial Ca^{2+} uptake and directly regulate oxidative phosphorylation and indirectly affect mitochondrial function by maintaining the mtDNA copy number and mitochondrial morphology [42]. Mutations in PKD1 and PKD2 lead to mitochondrial dysfunction and metabolic imbalance. Proinflammatory cytokine TNFα promote cyst formation, increased MCP-1 in cyst-lining cells and excretion of urinary MCP-1, and renal profibrotic macrophages in experimental ARPKD which might be associated with defects in mitophagy are also reported in patients with ADPKD. Loss of PC2 enhanced mitochondrial Ca^{2+} uptake, mitochondrial bioenergetics, and mitochondrial-ER tethering associated with increased Mfn2, and knockdown of Mfn2 rescued ER-dependent mitochondrial Ca^{2+} signaling are associated with reduced cyst proliferation [4]. Mitochondria of cyst-lining cells in the kidney of a mouse model of ADPKD display morphological abnormalities and decreased mtDNA. There is reduced peroxisome proliferator-activated receptor γ coactivator 1α (PGC-1α), which regulates mitochondrial biogenesis. Functional mitochondrial abnormalities and increased mROS production indicate that mitochondrial dysfunction plays a functional role in cystogenesis [4, 43].

4.1.4 Lupus nephritis

Renal involvement in systemic lupus erythematosus (SLE) occurs in 40–50% of adult patients, and results in end stage renal disease (ESRD) about 10% of patients despite modifications in therapeutic strategies [44]. LN is the most common severe manifestation of systemic lupus erythematosus. The pathogenesis of LN is multifactorial, and includes aberrant T-cell and B-cell signaling, autoantibody production, and deregulated cytokine secretion. Various genetic as well as environmental factors also contribute [45, 46]. The T-cells of SLE show increased mitochondrial mass (megamitochondria), mitochondrial hyper-polarization, and ATP depletion which lead to aberrant activation and enhanced necrosis of T-cells. This leads to release of extracellular mitochondria and their components and are recognized as damage-associated molecular patterns (DAMPs) that initiate innate and adaptive immune responses to elicit an inflammatory response that triggers organ damage [47]. Nitric oxide (NO)-dependent mitochondrial biogenesis could account for megamitochondria leading to sustained T-cell activation. On the other hand, increased T-cell mitochondria in SLE have also been attributed to insufficient mitophagy. Sequestration and successful clearance of damaged mitochondria by mitophagy suppresses mtROS accumulation, prevents inflammation and generation of autoantigens by intracellular oxidation suggesting that mitophagy is a potential therapeutic target for SLE and LN [46–48].

Gkirtzimanaki et al. observed that IFNα damages mitochondrial metabolism and mediates lysosomal dysfunction, impeding mitochondrial clearance and leading to cytosolic accumulation of mtDNA in monocytes [49]. Caspase-1 gets activated in the podocytes of both lupus nephritis patients and lupus-prone mice and inhibit mitophagy and amplify mitochondrial damage, mediated by cleavage of the key mitophagy regulator Parkin in lipopolysaccharide (LPS)-primed bone-marrow-derived macrophages [50].

Drp1, fusion mediator of mitochondria, is reduced in T cells from SLE patients and lupus-prone mice, concomitant with the accumulation of mitochondria.

Mitochondrial hyperpolarization and reactive oxygen intermediates production have been detected in peripheral blood T-lymphocytes from SLE patients, together with diminished levels of intracellular ATP, indicating dysfunction in mitochondria of T-cells in patients with lupus nephritis. CD4þT cells from SLE exhibit an increased mitochondrial mass and size due to increased mitochondrial biogenesis and defective mitophagy [51].

4.1.5 Membranous nephropathy & focal and segmental glomerulosclerosis

Membranous nephropathy (MN) is a most common cause of adult nephrotic syndrome. Various podocytic autoantigens have been implicated in the pathogenesis of the disease. Phospholipase A2 receptor (PLA2R) is the major autoantigen on podocytes in primary MN, whereas thrombospondin type-I domain-containing 7A (THSD7A) is the minor antigen, the antibodies to which are predominantly of the IgG4 subclass [52].

Cultured podocytes when exposed to sera from patients with MN revealed mitochondrial fragmentation, loss of membrane potential, and mROS production [53]. Patients with MN also show increased glomerular mitochondrial fission proteins, DRP1, phosphorylated-DRP1 (Ser-616), and FIS1. The observation of these studies show that podocytic injury in MN is secondary to mitochondrial dysfunction [53].

Focal segmental glomerular sclerosis (FSGS), also a common cause of nephrotic syndrome in pediatric as well as adults, is one of the major renal complication of mitochondrial cytopathies.

The mitochondrial DNA (mtDNA) encodes for 13 structural genes of OXPHOS enzymes, two ribosomal RNAs, and 22 transfer RNAs. Glomerular involvement of an A-to-G transition at mtDNA position 3243 in the gene for $tRNA^{Leu}$(UUR) has been implicated in FSGS. Recent studied with a mouse model carrying mutant mtDNA with a 4696-bp deletion, developed focal and segmental glomerulosclerosis and died within 6 months due to renal failure [54, 55].

Puromycin aminonucleoside nephrosis (PAN) model to study FSGS reveals reduction of respiratory chain enzymatic activities, oxygen consumption, and the swelling of renal tubular mitochondria [56]. Reduction of the intraglomerular mtDNA-encoded protein, COX I, suggests that there is either an induction of mtDNA damage or a reduction in mtDNA copy number during the progression of PAN. Several studies have described mitochondrial dysfunction and/or mtDNA changes in glomerular diseases like accumulation of oxidative damage of mtDNA in the kidney of streptozotocin-induced diabetes rats, and downregulation of respiratory chain complex in patients with the congenital nephrotic syndrome of the Finnish type [57].

MCs comprise one of the causes of primary FSGS, among which mitochondrial myopathy, encephalopathy, lactic acidosis, and stroke like episodes (MELAS) syndrome account for a large proportion. MELAS syndrome is mainly caused by point mutations in the *MTTL1* gene, encoding mitochondrial tRNALEU. Renal biopsies from patients with coexistence of MELAS and FSGS often manifest with numerous dysmorphic mitochondria in podocytes and effacement of foot processes [58].

4.1.6 Tubular defects and role of mitochondria

Renal tubules comprise one of the major victims of MCs, of which the most frequently reported is proximal tubular defects. Proximal tubular cells are relatively vulnerable to oxidative stress and are therefore apt to suffer from respiratory chain defects. Renal tubule defects mainly manifest as loss of electrolytes and low-molecular-weight proteins, which are frequently characterized as Fanconi syndrome and Bartter-like syndrome. Patients with mitochondrial tubulopathy are usually accompanied by myoclonic epilepsy and ragged red muscle fibers (MERRF), and Pearson's, Kearns-Sayre, and Leigh syndromes. The majority of genetic mutations detected in these diseases are fragment deletions of mtDNA [6, 7, 59–61].

4.1.7 Acute kidney injury (AKI)

AKI is defined as an abrupt (within hours) decrease in kidney function, which encompasses both injury (structural damage) and impairment (loss of function). AKI is common (8–16% of hospital admissions) and many aspects of its natural history remain uncertain [62]. Classification of AKI includes pre-renal AKI, acute post-renal obstructive nephropathy and intrinsic acute kidney diseases. Of these, only 'intrinsic' AKI represents true kidney disease, and the most common etiologies are toxins, ischemia, sepsis and obstructive injury [63]. Disruption of mitochondrial integrity in renal tubular cells is considered as the common findings in all forms of AKI [64]. In AKI, mitochondrial damage contributes critically to sublethal and lethal injury of kidney tubules, and the consequent loss of renal function. In various models of AKI, mitochondrial dynamics are disrupted, resulting in mitochondrial fragmentation, membrane permeabilization, mitochondrial dysfunction, energetic failure, and ROS production [9]. There is decreased antioxidant defenses, injured mitochondrial respiration, intrarenal inflammatory response and oxidative stress along with downregulation of protein expression during mitochondrial metabolism and decreased oxygen are seen [65]. Elevated mitochondrial DNA levels in the urine has been considered as a novel non-invasive biomarker for detecting mitochondrial dysfunction. Eirin et al. revealed that increased urinary mtDNA (UmtDNA) in hypertensive patients correlated with other biomarkers of renal dysfunction and glomerular hyperfiltration [66, 67]. Derangements of mitochondrial integrity may be associated with the detectable release of UmtDNA in sepsis-induced AKI has never been determined. Sepsis activates several pathological mechanisms linked to mitochondria, including hypoperfusion, oxidative stress, and the inflammatory response. Ultrastructural changes observed in the kidney tubular cells include mitochondrial impairment, swelling and cellular death. Disruption of mitochondrial integrity in the renal tubular epithelial cells leads to release of mitochondrial DAMPs into the urine which can be used as a surrogate biomarker of renal mitochondrial damage [68].

Expression of genes involved in oxidative phosphorylation are reduced as demonstrated by Parikh et al [69]. There is proportional decrease in expression of PGC-1a expression with reduction of renal function. Activation of PGC-1a promotes recovery from AKI caused by sepsis. cGAS–STING pathway activation is involved in autoimmune and inflammatory reactions, that activate by self-genomic DNA damage. Cyclic GMP–AMP synthase (cGAS) is a pattern recognition receptor that recognizes double-stranded DNA in the cytoplasm and then binds to the trans-membrane protein, a stimulator of interferon genes (STING) localized on the endoplasmic reticulum (ER). A relationship between mitochondrial damage and induction of cGAS–STING pathway in inflamed proximal tubular cells has been postulated in Cisplatin induced AKI. In ischemic and cisplatin nephrotoxic AKI, the fusion-fission mitochondrial dynamics in proximal tubules reveal that mitochondrial fission initiated by Drp1 occurs immediately after the injury [69–72].

4.1.7.1 Mitophagy and acute kidney injury

Recent literature suggests that mitophagy is involved in the pathophysiological processes of AKI. PINK1/Parkin-mediated mitophagy has a protective role for mitochondrial quality control in the context of tubular cell survival and function. Tang et al. demonstrated both PINK1 and Parkin are upregulated in renal tubular epithelial cells during ischemic AKI *in vitro* and *in vivo*, PINK1 and/or Parkin deficiency results in increased mitochondrial damage, ROS production, and inflammation causing increased tubular damage and aggravated AKI [73]. Boston University mouse proximal tubular cell line (BUPMT cells) show upregulation of BNIP3 following oxygen–glucose deprivation-reperfusion, and in kidney tissues of mouse models. BNIP3-deficient mice renal tubular epithelial cells show accumulation of damaged mitochondria, increased ROS production, enhanced cell apoptosis, and inflammation. These findings strongly support the involvement of multiple mitophagy regulatory pathways in the pathogenesis of AKI [74].

Wang et al. stated that Bax inhibitor-1 (BI1) promotes mitochondrial retention of PHB2 and improves mitophagy, preserving mitochondrial homeostasis in a murine AKI model. He also demonstrated that renal functional loss, tissue damage, and apoptosis are aggravated in cisplatin-treated *Pink1−/−* and *Parkin−/−* mice relative to cisplatin-treated wild-type mice, suggesting that activation of PINK1/Parkin-mediated mitophagy plays a protective role against cisplatin nephrotoxicity [3]. A recent study by Zhu et al. demonstrated that trehalose administration attenuates mitochondrial dysfunction through activating transcriptional factor EB (TFEB)-mediated autophagy and mitophagy in cisplatin-induced AKI *in vitro* and *in vivo*. The study sheds lights on the roles of TFEB on mitophagy and provides a novel promising therapeutic target for AKI [75].

Notably, preservation of mitochondrial dynamics, prevention of mitochondrial membrane permeabilization, and/or promotion of mitochondrial biogenesis can protect kidney tubular cells and tissues in AKI.

4.1.8 Tubulointerstitial fibrosis

Tubulointerstitial fibrosis follows following aberrant kidney repair following AKI, eventually progressing to CKD. Suppression of the proinflammatory cytokines interleukin (IL)-18 and IL-1β and nod-like receptor family pyrin domain containing 3 (NLRP3) inflammasome activation, inhibits progression to CKD following prolonged ischemia. Studies indicate that mitochondrial dysfunction plays a role in inflammation leading to tubulointerstitial fibrosis and development of end-stage renal disease. Analysis of genome-wide transcriptome-based analyses revealed that human fibrotic kidneys have lower expression of various mitochondrial enzymes and regulators of fatty acid oxidation along with higher intracellular lipid deposition. Fibrosis is mediated by monocyte chemoattractant protein 1 (MCP-1), a chemokine that promotes the infiltration of monocytes, inflammation, and fibrosis, the levels of which are increased with decreased renal expression of mitophagy regulators (PINK1, MFN2, and Parkin) in experimental and human kidney fibrosis. Mitophagy impairment led to an accumulation of abnormal mitochondria, augmented macrophage induced fibrotic response, superoxide production, and reduced ATP synthesis. Deficiency of mitophagy by Pink1 or Park2 gene deletion markedly increased mROS production and mitochondrial damage, which worsened renal fibrosis. These effects were rescued by a mitochondria-targeted antioxidant. Defective mitochondrial metabolism and reduced expression of mitophagy regulators have been shown to enhance the renal inflammatory and fibrotic responses and mediate the progression of CKD [4, 76–78].

Author details

Lovelesh K. Nigam*, Aruna V. Vanikar, Rashmi Dalsukhbhai Patel, Kamal V. Kanodia, Kamlesh Suthar and Umang Thakkar
Department of Pathology, Laboratory Medicine, Transfusion Services and Immunohematology, G.R. Doshi and K.M. Mehta Institute of Kidney Diseases and Research Centre and Dr. H.L. Trivedi Institute of Transplantation Sciences, Ahmedabad, India

*Address all correspondence to: drloveleshnigam@gmail.com

References

[1] Henze K, Martin W (November 2003). "Evolutionary biology: essence of mitochondria". *Nature*. 426 (6963): 127-128. Bibcode: 2003 Natur.426:127H. doi:10.1038/426127a. PMID 14614484. S2CID 862398.

[2] Siekevitz P (1957). "Powerhouse of the cell". *Scientific American*. 197 (1): 131-140. Bibcode:1957SciAm.197a.131S. doi:10.1038/scientificamerican0757-131.

[3] Wang Y, Cai J, Tang C, Dong Z. Mitophagy in Acute Kidney Injury and Kidney Repair. Cells 2020, 9, 338; doi:10.3390/cells9020338

[4] Bhatia D, Capili A, Choi ME. Mitochondrial dysfunction in kidney injury, inflammation, and disease: potential therapeutic approaches. Kidney Res Clin Pract 2020;39(3): 244-258; pISSN: 2211-9132,eISSN: 2211-9140:https://doi.org/10.23876/j.krcp.20.082

[5] Maezawa Y., Takemoto M., Yokote K. (2015). Cell biology of diabetic nephropathy: roles of endothelial cells, tubulointerstitial cells and podocytes. *J. Diabetes Investig.* 6, 3-15. 10.1111/jdi.12255, PMID: **25621126,** PMCID: PMC4296695, DOI: 10.1111/jdi.12255

[6] Che R,Yuan Y, Huang S, Zhang A. Mitochondrial dysfunction in the pathophysiology of renal diseases. *Am J Physiol Renal Physiol 2013;* 306: F367–F378: doi:10.1152/ajprenal.00571.2013.

[7] Eirin A. The Emerging Role of Mitochondrial Targeting in Kidney Disease. Hand b Exp Pharmacol. 2017 ; 240: 229-250. doi:10.1007/164_2016_6.

[8] Nowak G. Protein kinase C-alpha and ERK1/2 mediate mitochondrial dysfunction, decreases in active Na+ transport, and cisplatin-induced apoptosis in renal cells. J Biol Chem 2002;277:43377-43388.

[9] Govers LP, Toka HR, Hariri A, Walsh SB, Bockenhauer D. Mitochondrial DNA mutations in renal disease: an overview. Pediatric Nephrology 2020;36:9-17: https://doi.org/10.1007/s00467-019-04404-6

[10] Nicolson GL. Mitochondrial Dysfunction and chronic disease: Treatment with natural supplements. Integrative Medicine 2014;13(4):35-43.

[11] Mishra P, Chan DC. Mitochondrial dynamics and inheritance during cell division, development and disease. Nat Rev Mol Cell Biol 2014;15:634-646.

[12] Bhargava P, Schnellmann RG. Mitochondrial energetics in the kidney. Nat Rev Nephrol 2017;13:629-646.

[13] Zhan M, Brooks C, Liu F, Sun L, Dong Z. Mitochondrial dynamics: regulatory mechanisms and emerging role in renal pathophysiology. Kidney Int 2013;83:568-581.

[14] Twig G, Shirihai OS. The interplay between mitochondrial dynamics and mitophagy. Antioxid Redox Signal. 2011;14(10:1939-1951.

[15] Zuo Z, Jing K, Wu H, Wang S, Ye L, Li Z, Yang C, Pan Q, Liu WJ and Liu H-f (2020) Mechanisms and Functions of Mitophagy and Potential Roles in Renal Disease.Front. Physiol. 11:935.doi: 10.3389/fphys.2020.00935

[16] Zhan M, Brooks C, Liu F, Sun L, Dong Z. Mitochondrial dynamics: regulatory mechanisms and emerging

role in renal pathophysiology. Kidney International 2013:83;568-81.

[17] Ishimoto Y, Inagi R. Mitochondria: a therapeutic target in acute kidney injury. Nephrol Dial Transplant 2016;31: 1062-1069:doi:10.11093/ndt/gfv317.

[18] Tang C, He L, Liu J, Dong Z. Mitophagy: Basic mechanism and potential role in kidney diseases. Kidney Dis 2015;1:71-79:DOI:10.1159/000381510.

[19] Galvan DL, Green NH, Danesh FR. The hallmarks of mitochondrial dysfunction in chronic kidney disease. Kidney Int. 2017;92(5):1051-1057. doi:10.1016/j.kint.2017.05.034.

[20] Palikaras K, Lionaki E, Tavernarakis N. Mechanisms of mitophagy in cellular homeostasis, physiology and pathology. Nat Cell Biol. 2018 Sep;20(9):1013-1022. doi: 10.1038/s41556-018-0176-2. Epub 2018 Aug 28. PMID: 30154567.

[21] Sun N, Yun J, Liu J, et al. Measuring In Vivo Mitophagy. *Mol Cell*. 2015;60(4):685-696. doi:10.1016/j.molcel.2015.10.009.

[22] Chen M, Chen Z, Wang Y, Tan Z, Zhu C, Li Y, Han Z, Chen L, Gao R, Liu L, Chen Q. Mitophagy receptor FUNDC1 regulates mitochondrial dynamics and mitophagy. Autophagy. 2016;12(4):689-702. doi: 10.1080/15548627.2016.1151580. PMID: 27050458; PMCID: PMC4836026.

[23] Choi, G.E., Lee, H.J., Chae, C.W. *et al.* BNIP3L/NIX-mediated mitophagy protects against glucocorticoid-induced synapse defects. *Nat Commun* **12,** 487 (2021). https://doi.org/10.1038/s41467-020-20679-y

[24] Bhujabal Z, Birgisdottir ÅB, Sjøttem E, Brenne HB, Øvervatn A, Habisov S, Kirkin V, Lamark T, Johansen T. FKBP8 recruits LC3A to mediate Parkin-independent mitophagy. EMBO Rep. 2017 Jun;18(6):947-961. doi: 10.15252/embr.201643147. Epub 2017 Apr 5. PMID: 28381481; PMCID: PMC5452039.

[25] Zhou, R., Yazdi, A., Menu, P. *et al.* A role for mitochondria in NLRP3 inflammasome activation. *Nature* **469,** 221-225 (2011). https://doi.org/10.1038/nature09663.

[26] USRDS: United States Renal Data System Annual Data Report:Epidemiology of Kidney Disease in the United States, Bethesda,MD, National Institute of Diabetes and Digestive and Kidney Diseases, 2015.

[27] Reutens AT: Epidemiology of diabetic kidney disease. Med Clin North Am 97: 1-18, 2013.

[28] World Health Organization: Global Status Report on Noncommunicable Diseases, Geneva, Switzerland, World Health Organization, 2014.

[29] Kwak SH, Park KS, Lee KU, Lee HK. Mitochondrial metabolism and diabetes. *J Diabetes Investig*. 2010;1(5):161-169. doi:10.1111/j.2040-1124.2010.00047.x

[30] Coughlan MT, Higgins GC, Tuong-Vi Nguyen, Penfold SA, Thallas-Bonke V, Tan SM, et al. Deficiency in Apoptosis-Inducing Factor Recapitulates Chronic Kidney Disease via Aberrant Mitochondrial Homeostasis. Diabetes Apr 2016, 65 (4) 1085-1098; DOI: 10.2337/db15-0864.

[31] Gao CL, Zhu C, Zhao YP, Chen XH, Ji CB, Zhang CM, Zhu JG, Xia ZK, Tong ML, Guo XR. Mitochondrial dysfunction is induced by high levels of glucose and free fatty acids in 3T3-L1 adipocytes. Mol Cell Endocrinol.

2010 May 14;320(1-2):25-33. doi: 10.1016/j.mce.2010.01.039. Epub 2010 Feb 6. PMID: 20144685.

[32] Xiao L, Xu X, Zhang F, et al. The mitochondria-targeted antioxidant MitoQ ameliorated tubular injury mediated by mitophagy in diabetic kidney disease via Nrf2/PINK1. Redox Biol 2017;11:297-311.

[33] Higgins GC, Coughlan MT. Mitochondrial dysfunction and mitophagy: the beginning and end to diabetic nephropathy? Br J Pharmacol. 2014 Apr;171(8):1917-42. doi: 10.1111/bph.12503. PMID: 24720258; PMCID: PMC3976613.

[34] Pinti MV, Fink GK, Hathaway QA, Durr AJ, Kunovac A, Hollander JM. Mitochondrial dysfunction in type 2 diabetes mellitus: an organ-based analysis. Am J Physiol Endocrinol Metab 2019;316:E268–E285; doi:10.1152/ajpendo.00314.2018.

[35] Wei PZ, Kwan BC, Chow KM, et al. Urinary mitochondrial DNA level is an indicator of intra-renal mitochondrial depletion and renal scarring in diabetic nephropathy.Nephrol Dial Transplant 2018;33:784-788.

[36] Coughlan MT, Thorburn DR, Penfold SA, et al. RAGEinduced cytosolic ROS promote mitochondrial superoxide generation in diabetes. J Am Soc Nephrol 2009;20:742-752.

[37] Rodrigues JC, Haas M, Reich HN. IgA nephropathy. Clin J Am Soc Nephrol 2017;12:677-686.

[38] Kiryluk K, Moldoveanu Z, Sanders JT, Eison TM, Suzuki H, Julian BA, et al. Aberrant glycosylation of IgA1 is inherited in both paediatric IgA nephropathy and Henoch-Schönlein purpura nephritis. *Kidney Int***80***:* 79-87, 2011.

[39] Nishida M, Morimoto M, Ohno K, Hamaoka K. IgA nephropathy in a girl with mitochondrial disease. Pediatr Int 2015;57:e50-e52.

[40] Bhreathnach U, Griffin B, Brennan E, Ewart L, Higgins D, Murphy M. Profibrotic IHG-1 complexes with renal disease associated HSPA5 and TRAP1 in mitochondria. Biochim Biophys Acta Mol Basis Dis 2017;1863:896-906.

[41] Igarashi P, Somlo S. Genetics and Pathogenesis of Polycystic kidney disease. JASN 2002. 13(9) 2384-2398;doi:http://doi.org/10.1097/01.ASN0000028643.17901.42.

[42] Padovano V, Podrini C, Boletta A, Caplan MJ. Metabolism and mitochondria in polycystic kidney disease research and therapy. Nat Rev Nephrol 2018;14:678-687.

[43] Ishimoto Y, Inagi R, Yoshihara D, et al. Mitochondrial abnormality facilitates cyst formation in autosomal dominant polycystic kidney disease. Mol Cell Biol 2017;37:e00337-17.

[44] Salama AD, Caplin B. Lupus Nephritis and Chronic Kidney Disease. The Journal of Rheumatology. **2020, 47** (9) 1303-1304; DOI: https://doi.org/10.3899/jrheum.200566.

[45] Liu Y. Anders H.-J. Lupus Nephritis: From Pathogenesis to Targets for Biologic Treatment. Nephron Clin Pract 2014;128:224-231. https://doi.org/10.1159/000368581

[46] Becker Y, Loignon RC, Julien AS, Marcoux G, Allaeys I, Lévesque T, et al. Anti-mitochondrial autoantibodies in systemic lupus erythematosus and their association with disease manifestations. Scientific reports. (2019) 9:4530. https://doi.org/10.1038/s41598-019-40900-3.

[47] Zhang C, Wang H, Yin L, Mao Y, Zhou W. Immunometabolism in the pathogenesis of systemic lupus erythematosus. Journal of Translational Autoimmunity. Journal of Translational Autoimmunity 3 (2020) 100046

[48] Minton K. Inflammasome: anti-inflammatory effect of mitophagy. *Nat. Rev. Immunol.* 2016;**16**:206-206.

[49] Gkirtzimanaki K, Kabrani E, Nikoleri D, et al. IFNα Impairs Autophagic Degradation of mtDNA Promoting Autoreactivity of SLE Monocytes in a STING-Dependent Fashion. *Cell Rep*. 2018;25(4):921-933.e5. doi:10.1016/j.celrep.2018.09.001

[50] Geisler S., Holmström K.M., Skujat D., Fiesel F.C., Rothfuss O.C., Kahle P.J., Springer W. PINK1/Parkin-mediated mitophagy is dependent on VDAC1 and p62/SQSTM1. *Nat. Cell Biol.* 2010;**12**:119-131.

[51] T.N. Caza, G. Talaber, A. Perl, Metabolic regulation of organelle homeostasis in lupus T cells, Clin. Immunol. 144 (2012) 200-213, https://doi.org/10.1016/ j.clim.2012.07.001.

[52] Xu Z, Chen L, Xiang H, Zhang C, Xiong J. Advances in Pathogenesis of Idiopathic Membranous Nephropathy. Kidney Dis 2020;6:330-345. https://doi.org/10.1159/000507704

[53] Buelli S, Perico L, Galbusera M, et al. Mitochondrial dependent autoimmunity in membranous nephropathy of IgG4-related disease. E Bio Medicine 2015;2:456-466.

[54] Lim K, Steele D, Fenves A, Thadhani R, Heher E, Karaa A. Focal segmental glomerulosclerosis associated with mitochondrial disease. *Clin Nephrol Case Stud*. 2017;5:20-25. Published 2017 Mar 3. doi:10.5414/CNCS109083

[55] Dinour D, Mini S, Polak-Charcon S, Lotan D, Holtzman EJ. Progressive nephropathy associated with mitochondrial tRNA gene mutation. Clin Nephrol. 2004; 62:149-154. [PubMed: 15356973]

[56] Hagiwara M, Yamagata K, Capaldi RA, Koyama A. Mitochondrial dysfunction in focal segmental glomerulosclerosis of puromycin aminonucleoside nephrosis. Kidney Int. 2006 Apr;69(7):1146-52. doi: 10.1038/sj.ki.5000207. PMID: 16609681.

[57] Holthofer H, Kretzler M, Haltia A, et al. Altered gene expression and functions of mitochondria in human nephrotic syndrome. *FASEB.* 1999; 13: 523-532

[58] Hanna MG, Nelson IP, Morgan-Hughes JA, *et al.* MELAS: a new disease associated mitochondrial DNA mutation and evidence for further genetic heterogeneity. *Journal of Neurology, Neurosurgery & Psychiatry* 1998;**65:**512-517.

[59] Lee YS, Yap HK, Barshop BA, Lee YS, Rajalingam S, Loke KY. Mitochondrial tubulopathy: the many faces of mitochondrial disorders. Pediatr Nephrol. 2001 Sep;16(9):710-2. doi: 10.1007/s004670100637. PMID: 11511982.

[60] Francesco Emma, Giovanni Montini, Leonardo Salviati, Carlo Dionisi-Vici, "Renal Mitochondrial Cytopathies", *International Journal of Nephrology*, vol. 2011, Article ID 609213, 10 pages, 2011. https://doi.org/10.4061/2011/609213

[61] Finsterer J and Finsterer J: Renal manifestations of primary mitochondrial disorders (Review). Biomed Rep 6: 487-494, 2017.

[62] Sawhney S, Marks A, Fluck N, Levin A, Prescott G.J., Black C.

Intermediate and long-term outcomes of survivors of acute kidney injury episodes: a large population-based cohort study. *Am J Kidney Dis.* 2017;69: 18-28. http://dx.doi.org/10.1053/j.ackd.2017.05.001

[63] Konstantinos Makris, Loukia Spanou. Acute Kidney Injury: Definition, Pathophysiology and Clinical Phenotypes. Clin Biochem Rev. 2016 May; 37(2): 85-98. PMCID: PMC5198510. PMID: 28303073

[64] S. M. Parikh, Y. Yang, L. He, C. Tang, M. Zhan, and Z. Dong, "Mitochondrial function and disturbances in the septic kidney," Seminars in Nephrology, 35(1):pp. 108-119, 2015.

[65] J. Hinkelbein, L. Böhm, S. Braunecker, C. Adler, E. De Robertis, and F. Cirillo, "Decreased tissue COX5B expression and mitochondrial dysfunction during sepsis-induced kidney injury in rats," Oxidative Medicine and Cellular Longevity, vol. 2017, Article ID 8498510, 24 pages, 2017.

[66] A. Eirin, A. Saad, H. Tang et al., "Urinary mitochondrial DNA copy number identifies chronic renal injury in hypertensive patients," Hypertension, vol. 68, no. 2, pp. 401-410, 2016.

[67] A. Eirin, A. Saad, J. R. Woollard et al., "Glomerular hyperfiltration in obese African American hypertensive patients is associated with elevated urinary mitochondrial-DNA copy number," American Journal of Hypertension, vol. 30, no. 11, pp. 1112-1119, 2017.

[68] Qiongyuan Hu ,1 Jianan Ren ,1 Huajian Ren,1 Jie Wu,1 Xiuwen Wu ,1 Song Liu ,2 Urinary Mitochondrial DNA Identifies Renal Dysfunction and Mitochondrial Damage in Sepsis-Induced Acute Kidney Injury. Oxidative Medicine and Cellular Longevity 2018; Article ID 8074936: https://doi.org/10.1155/2018/8074936

[69] Parikh S, Goldstein A, Koenig MK, Scaglia F, Enns GM, Saneto R, et al. Diagnosis and management of mitochondrial disease: a consensus statement from the Mitochondrial Medicine Society. Genet Med. 2015 Sep;17(9):689-701. doi: 10.1038/gim.2014.177. Epub 2014 Dec 11. PMID: 25503498; PMCID: PMC5000852.

[70] Chen Y, Zhou Z, Min W. Mitochondria, Oxidative Stress and Innate Immunity. *Front Physiol*. 2018;9:1487. Published 2018 Oct 18. doi:10.3389/fphys.2018.01487.

[71] Maekawa H, Inoue T, Ouchi H, Jao TM, Inoue R, Nishi H, Fujii R, Ishidate F, Tanaka T, Tanaka Y, Hirokawa N, Nangaku M, Inagi R. Mitochondrial Damage Causes Inflammation via cGAS-STING Signaling in Acute Kidney Injury. Cell Rep. 2019 Oct 29;29(5):1261-1273.e6. doi: 10.1016/j.celrep.2019.09.050. PMID: 31665638.

[72] Brooks C, Wei Q, Cho SG, Dong Z. Regulation of mitochondrial dynamics in acute kidney injury in cell culture and rodent models. J Clin Invest. 2009 May;119(5):1275-85. doi: 10.1172/JCI37829. Epub 2009 Apr 6. PMID: 19349686; PMCID: PMC2673870.

[73] Tang Z, Takahashi Y, He H, et al. TOM40 Targets Atg2 to Mitochondria-Associated ER Membranes for Phagophore Expansion. *Cell Rep*. 2019;28(7):1744-1757.e5. doi:10.1016/j.celrep.2019.07.036.

[74] Tang C, Han H, Liu Z, et al. Activation of BNIP3-mediated mitophagy protects against renal ischemia-reperfusion injury. *Cell Death Dis*. 2019;10(9):677. Published 2019 Sep 12. doi:10.1038/s41419-019-1899-0.

[75] Zhu L, Yuan Y, Yuan L, et al. Activation of TFEB-mediated autophagy by trehalose attenuates mitochondrial dysfunction in cisplatin-induced acute kidney injury. *Theranostics*. 2020;10(13):5829-5844. Published 2020 Apr 27. doi:10.7150/thno.44051.

[76] Qin J, Peng ZZ, Li Q, Wen R, Tao LJ. Renal Fibrosis and Mitochondrial Damage. *Chin Med J (Engl)*. 2018;131(22):2769-2772. doi:10.4103/0366-6999.245272

[77] Li, X., Zhang, W., Cao, Q. *et al.* Mitochondrial dysfunction in fibrotic diseases. *Cell Death Discov.* **6,** 80 (2020). https://doi.org/10.1038/s41420-020-00316-9.

[78] Jiang M, Mi Bai, Lei J, Xie Y, Xu S, Jia Z, et al. Mitochondrial dysfunction and the AKI-to-CKD transition. American Journal of Physiology-Renal Physiology 2020; 319(6):F1105-F1116:https://doi.org/10.1152/ajprenal.00285.2020.

Chapter 4

Maneuvering Mitochondria for Better Understanding of Therapeutic Potential of mtDNA Mutation

Sanket Tembe

Abstract

Heterogeneity of mitochondrial diseases in terms of genetic etiology and clinical management makes their diagnosis challenging. Mitochondrial genome, basic mitochondrial genetics, common mutations, and their correlation with human diseases is well-established now and advances in sequencing is accelerating the molecular diagnostics of mitochondrial diseases. Major research focus now is on development of mtDNA intervention techniques like mtDNA gene editing, transfer of exogenous genes (sometimes even entire mtDNA) that would compensate for mtDNA mutations responsible for mitochondrial dysfunction. Although these genetic manipulation techniques have good potential for treatment of mtDNA diseases, research on such mitochondrial manipulation fosters ethical issues. The present chapter starts with an introduction to the factors that influence the clinical features of mitochondrial diseases. Advancement in treatments for mitochondrial diseases are then discussed followed by a note on methods for preventing transmission of these diseases.

Keywords: mitochondrial diseases, mtDNA intervention techniques, mitochondrial donation, genomics advancements, reproductive techniques

1. Introduction

Mitochondria are synonymized with energy thanks to their ability to produce most of the Adenosine Triphosphate (ATP) through the process of Oxidative Phosphorylation. In addition to ATP production, several metabolic processes like tricarboxylic acid cycle (TCA), fatty acid oxidation, ketogenesis, urea cycle (partly), heme and phospholipid synthesis take place in mitochondria [1, 2]. Role of mitochondria in cell death (apoptosis) is also well-established [3]. Recent research suggests new role of mitochondria in calcium homeostasis, iron and copper metabolism and inflammation and immunity [4]. Though oxidative phosphorylation puts aerobes at higher level in terms of efficiency of energy production, one unpleasant consequence of this important process is production of reactive oxygen species (ROS) also known as mitochondrial ROS (mtROS). The culprit for formation of these reactive species is proton leak at the inner mitochondrial membrane. Formation of such species pose great threat to mitochondrial DNA (mtDNA) and may lead to mitochondrial dysfunction [5]. Once thought to be uncommon, mtDNA diseases are now known to be quite prevalent and their definition is no more restricted to defects in oxidative phosphorylation alone but also include defects in molecular processes like mitochondrial fission, fusion and translation [6–8].

The list of common mitochondrial diseases and syndromes is quite lengthy that include mitochondrial encephalopathy, lactic acidosis and stroke-like episodes (MELAS syndrome), Leber's hereditary optic neuropathy (LHON), myoclinic epilepsy with ragged-red fibers (MERRF), Leigh syndrome and Pearson syndrome, Kearne-Sayre syndrome (KSS), chronic progressive external ophthalmoloplegia (CPEO) and neuropathy, ataxia and retinitis pigmentosa (NARP) [9–17]. Mutations in the mitochondrially-encoded genes are the most common cause of these diseases. Several mutations have been reported such as m.3243A > G, m.3271 T > C, m.1642G > A, m.9957 T > C, m.3272 T > C, m.1642G > A, m.1277A > G, m.13045A > C, m.13513G > A and m.13514A > G (all reported in MELAS [18–26]), m.8344A > G, m.8356G > A, m.3291 T > C, m.4279A > G (reported in MERRF [27–29]), G3460A, T14484C in LHON [30]. Recent review describes a comprehensive approach to study mitochondrial disorders caused by mutations through an example of m.3243 A > G [31].

Reviews on basic mitochondrial genetics, mutations and their correlation with human diseases are available [32–34]. Starting with unique features of mitochondria that decide the clinical presentation of mitochondrial diseases, this review focusses on advancement in mitochondrial DNA manipulation. Methods for preventing transmission of these diseases are discussed at the end.

2. Factors that govern clinical features of mitochondrial diseases

2.1 Heteroplasmy

Presence of several thousand copies of mitochondrial genome (mtGenome) per cell creates two conditions; homoplasmy and heteroplasmy. When all copies of mtGenome are identical, the scenario is described as homoplasmy. Heteroplasmy is a situation in which more than one mtDNA variants exist between the cells of an individual or within a same cell. Often this is due to de novo mutations either in germ line or in somatic cells. As a result, mitochondrial dysfunction can be seen only in specific cells, tissues, or organs. The rate at which the regions in the mtGenome evolves is much higher than that of nuclear genes. This reduces the possibility of all mtDNA molecules to be identical in an individual's cells. Considering the large copy number of mtGenome present, detection of mtDNA mutation is difficult until it is spread among enough mtDNA molecules in a given cell. Only when mutated mtDNA exceeds threshold levels, clinical consequences of such mutations are seen [35]. Absence of fixed functional threshold level makes the analysis of mtDNA results even more complicated. Variations in threshold frequencies have been reported for different types of tissues and mtDNA mutations.

2.2 Mitochondrial DNA bottleneck

Mitochondrial genome, unlike its nuclear counterpart, shows uniparental transmission. Considering a single-parent origin, theoretically, mitochondrial DNA of a mother and her progeny should not show any variations. But, in reality, extensive variations have been reported in humans [36, 37]. Accumulation and enrichment of mutant mitochondria thus suggests presence of mitochondrial bottleneck; a concept that describes why mtDNA of an embryo may differ significantly from that of its mother [38].

3. Manipulation of mitochondrial DNA

Diagnosis and monitoring clinical progression of mtDNA diseases is difficult due to multi-copy nature of mtGenome. Fortunately, many harmful mtDNA mutations are heteroplasmic and this paves the way for curing these disorders. If mutated copies of mtDNAmolecules can be removed selectively from the pool of wild type molecules, heteroplasmy can be reduced and cellular biochemical defects can be cured. However, manipulating heteroplasmy has been challenging due to several barriers. Some of these barriers and attempts to overcome them are discussed in this section.

3.1 First barrier: difficulty in mitochondrial transfection

Mitochondria have two lipid bilayers that includes outer and inner membranes. While outer membrane allows easy transport of small molecules like ATP, proteins less than 10 KDaand ions, the inner mebrane brings selectivity barrier. Hydrophilic molecules cannot cross this barrier due to presence of cardiolipin; a hallmark mitochondrial lipid with four alkyl tails. It is this impermeability of inner membrane to the hydrophilic molecules that makes the passage of DNA through mitochondrial membranes difficult.

3.2 Strategies to overcome mitochondrial membrane barrier

One of the effective ways to treat mitochondrial diseases is to introduce wild type genes into the mitochondria. The approaches for introducing genes can be broadly classified into three categories namely physical, chemical, and biological methods. Physical methods are relatively simple and straightforward. Methods like microinjection, particle bombardment, electroporation and sonication have been used for delivering exogenous genes into the mitochondria [39, 40]. Separate carrier molecules are not required in these methods which eliminates the toxicity problems of such molecules. However, drawbacks of these methods include random distribution of DNA in mitochondrial matrix and the risk of damage of target cell during cell membrane penetration [40].

Many chemical-based methods have been reported for mitochondrial gene delivery. Considering hydrophobicity and presence of negative charges on mitochondrial membrane, cationic and amphiphilic carrier molecules have been used to enclose the negatively charged DNA [41]. Plasmid DNA was introduced to mitochondria using rhodamine-pDNA-nanoparticle complex [42] where the dye facilitated movement of nanoparticles across the plasma membrane and mitochondrial membrane. Mitochondria-specific liposomes were used for successful release of plasmid DNA in mitochondrial matrix [43], however, certain limitations like cytotoxicity and low transfection efficiency were noted. Improved version of liposome-based nanocarrier came in the form of MITO-Porter [44, 45]. Current research focuses on improving the mitochondrial targeting and reducing the toxicity to target cells. New ligands are being explored and linked to chemically synthesized carrier molecules that target the mitochondrial receptors.

Understanding of mitochondrial targeting signal peptide (MTS)-mediated translocation has provided a new biological approach for specific mitochondrial gene delivery. Carrier molecules having DNA-binding ability were conjugated to MTS. DNA oligomer peptide nucleic acid (PNA) that has polyamide bond rather than usual sugar-phosphate backbone, was conjugated to MTS and this MTS-mediated PNA could successfully enter the mitochondrial matrix through the translocase of outer membrane (TOM) and that of inner membrane (TIM) [46, 47]. Though this approach has some shortcomings like low mitochondrial targeting (as PNA tends to be localized in nucleus) and the restricted size of genes-to be-transferred, this is a clear indication that MTS can be successfully applied in mitogene delivery in near future. Use of viral vectors, especially adeno-associated virus (AAV), have been tested for mitochondrial gene delivery [48]. The wild type human mitochondrial genes were added to MTS-AAV complex to compensate mutated and defective NADH ubiquinone oxidoreductase subunit 4 (ND4) gene which is the culprit for LHON [49]. In addition to these physical, chemical, and biological methods, there are several combinatorial approaches that have been tested. A recent review [50] gives details of these methods and also discusses the need for new approaches.

3.3 Barrier 2: eliminating mutant mtDNA molecules

Elimination of mutant mtDNA molecules can reduce the threshold of mutant molecule load. Total elimination of mutant mtDNA is not required because a small reduction in mutant mtDNA load just below the threshold can improve the clinical scenario of a diseased person.

3.4 Strategies to selectively target mutant molecules

Construction and characterization of mitoApaLI; one of the several mitochondria-targeted restriction endonucleases developed so far, and its significant role in shifting heteroplasmy towards one of the two mtDNA haplotypes is explained in detail in a recent book chapter [51]. The prerequisite (also a limiting factor) of using mitoREs is that the target mutation should result in a unique restriction site to avoid breaking of wild type mtDNA. Different methods of mitochondrial transfection and strategies to deal with heteroplasmy are summerized in **Figure 1.**

Two recent gene editing systems namely mitochondria-targeted transcription activator-like effector nucleases (mitoTALENs) and mitochondria-targeted zinc finger nucleases (mtZFN) can selectively target single nucleotide mutations and can degrade them. Minczuk and Gammage laboratories have extensively used mtZFN to shift heteroplasmy [52, 53]. The mitoTALENs have been used to target specific mutations from animal and human-derived cells [54]. Although these gene therapy approaches are quite promising, we need to be careful because of the risk involved in this approach. mtDNA copy number may go down significantly and there may be undesirable off-target effects while attempting elimination of mutated copies. Crisper-Cas 9 cannot be used for this purpose because it needs single-guide RNA for gene editing and RNA import in mitochondria is restricted [55].

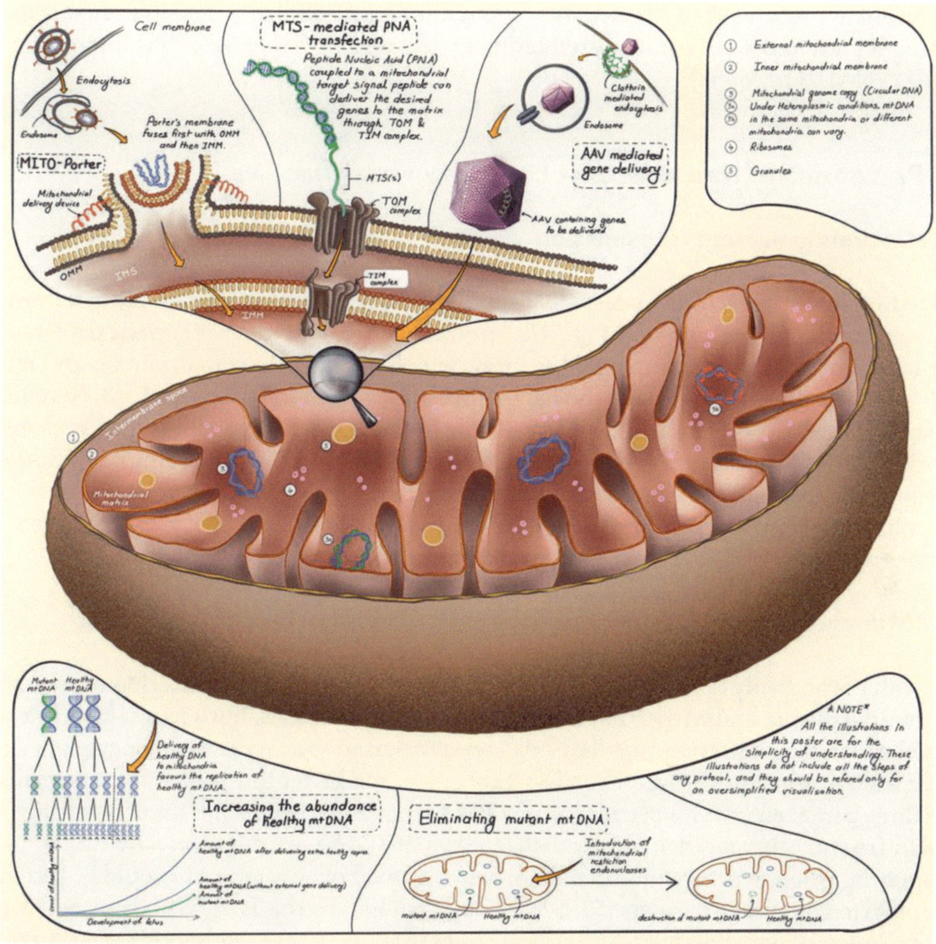

Figure 1.
The figure is a schematic representation of different methods of mitochondrial transfection and strategies to deal with heteroplasmy. Abbreviations used in the figure are: Outer mitochondrial membrane (OMM), intermembrane space (IMS), inner mitochondrial membrane (IMM), mitochondrial target signal peptide (MTS), translocase of outer membrane (TOM), translocase of inner membrane (TIM), adeno-associated virus (AAV) and mitochondrial DNA (mtDNA).

4. Decrease in NAD^+ levels

Nicotinamide adenine dinucleotide oxidized (NAD^+) is a coenzyme required for action of many enzymes like polyADP ribose polymerase (PARP) and sirtuin deacetylases. Substantial decrease in NAD^+concentration and the ratio of NAD^+/NADH was reported in the cells having defective mitochondria [56]. Defective respiratory chain cannot reoxidize NADH to oxygen. This results in reduction of pyruvate to lactate by lactate dehydrogenase generating NAD^+. Transport of excess lactate outside the cell leads to lactate acidemia, which is a common feature of mitochondrial diseases. Increasing the cellular levels of NAD^+ either through supplementation or through bringing changes in enzymes involved in its synthesis have been reported [57].

A recent approach tested in mice was to reoxidize extracellular lactate to pyruvate and bring it back to the cell for its re-reduction by lactate dehydrogenase thus increasing $NAD^+/NADH$ ratio [58].

5. Prevention of transmission of mitochondrial diseases

5.1 Options to prevent transmission

Mitochondrial DNA is maternally inherited and genetic bottleneck makes it even more peculiar. Therefore, options different from those with nuclear genetic defects must be considered. It is important to know which mutation a woman carries and its level; especially in those cases who harbor heteroplasmic mtDNA mutations. Genetic diagnosis and expert counseling is invaluable for such cases. Post-counseling options include voluntary childlessness and adoption. Prenatal testing and preimplantation genetic diagnosis (PGD) are recently available alternatives. PGD includes in vitro fertilization (IVF) and embryo development to blastocyst stage. Because of inherent issues with IVF, PGD has limited chance to succeed.

5.2 Mitochondrial replacement therapy (MRT) or mitochondrial donation

MRT is probably the only way available to those couples who are suffering from mitochondrial disease and wish to have a healthy child. In such cases, nucleus is taken from a mother carrying defective mitochondria and transferred to an enucleated oocyte or egg of a woman with healthy mitochondria. Embryo formed after this procedure (also called as three parent embryo) will have nuclear DNA from both parents but mitochondrial DNA from another mother. Ideally such embryo should be free from defective mitochondria. Using this technique in human oocytes, good quality embryos could be formed as reported by several workers [59, 60]. Though potentially this is a great advancement, mitochondrial donation may raise ethical issues [61]. Also some workers observed that the nucleus which was transferred to enucleated oocyte/egg showed presence of contaminating defective mitochondria. Enrichment of such contaminating mitochondria may cause mitochondrial disease in individuals generated through MRT. This issue becomes more sensitive when female embryos are generated after MRT because they will be passing on their defective mitochondria to the next generation. MRT females may show same mitochondrial disease and infertility as their mothers. In future, better understanding of maternal inheritance of mitochondria will improve the efficacy of this therapeutic method and make it a sustainable approach for betterment of individuals across the generations. Another issue that may hamper the progress of mitochondrial donation is availability of oocyte donors because this involves hormonal treatment.

6. Conclusions

Advances in DNA sequencing are accelerating the diagnosis of mitochondrial diseases and helping in assessment of heteroplasmy levels. Although molecular diagnosis is crucial, it can only identify the problem but cannot solve it. Input from reproductive biologists are equally important for comprehensive analysis and personal care of diseased individuals. Development of new treatments through further advancements in gene therapy holds great promise for the sufferers of mitochondrial disease.

Acknowledgements

I am grateful to the Principal, Fergusson College (Autonomous) and Head, Department of Biotechnology, Fergusson College for their support. I thank my colleague Monica Joshi for her help in proofreading the manuscript. I am thankful to my friend Mithila Shukla from Purdue University for sending me research articles. I also thank my undergraduate student Hrishikesh Hardikar for his help in preparing illustration and in formatting-related work.

Author details

Sanket Tembe
Department of Biotechnology, Fergusson College (Autonomous), Pune, India

*Address all correspondence to: sankettembe@fergusson.edu

References

[1] Nelson D, Cox M. Lehninger Principles of Biochemistry, 8th ed. W. H. Freeman, 2021.

[2] Voet D, Voet J, Pratt C. Fundamentals of Biochemistry: Life at the Molecular Level, 5thed. Wiley, 2016.

[3] Alberts B, Johnson A, Lewis J, Morgan D, Raff M, Roberts K, Walter P. Molecular Biology of The Cell, 6th ed. Garland Science, 2014.

[4] Prasun P. Mitochondrial Medicine: A Primer for Health Care Providers and Translational Researchers, 1st ed. Academic Press, Elsevier, 2019. DOI: 10.1016/C2018-0-01187-1

[5] Nissanka N, Moraes CT. Mitochondrial DNA damage and reactive oxygen species in neurodegenerative disease. FEBS Letters. 2018;592:728-742. DOI: 10.1002/1873-3468.12956

[6] Craven L, Alston CL, Taylor RW, Turnbull DM. Recent advances in mitochondrial disease. Annu. Rev. Genomic. Hum. Genet. 2017;18:257-275. DOI: 10.1146/annurev-genom-091416-035426

[7] Scarpelli M, Todeschini A, Volonghi I, Padovani A, Filosto M. Mitochondrial diseases: Advanced and issues. Appl. Clin. Genet. 2017;10:21-26. DOI: 10.2147/TACG.S94267

[8] Vafai SB, Mootha VK. Mitochondrial disorders as windows into an ancient organelle. Nature. 2012;491:374-383. DOI: 10.1038/nature11707

[9] El-Hattab AW, Adesina AM, Jones J, Scaglia F. MELAS syndrome: Clinical manifestations, pathogenesis, and treatment options. Mol. Genet. Metab. 2015;116:4-12. DOI: 10.1016/j.ymgme.2015.06.004

[10] Tuppen HA, Blakely EL, Turnbull DM, Taylor RW. Mitochondrial DNA mutations and human disease. Biochim.Biophys. Acta. 2010;1797(2):113-28. DOI: 10.1016/j.bbabio.2009.09.005

[11] Hirano M. Weighing in on Leber hereditary optic neuropathy: effects of mitochondrial mass. Brain. 2014 Feb;137(Pt 2):308-9. DOI: 10.1093/brain/awu005

[12] Craven L, Alston CL, Taylor RW, Turnbull DM. Recent advances in mitochondrial disease. Annu. Rev. Genomic. Hum. Genet. 2017;18:257-275. DOI: 10.1146/annurev-genom-091416-035426

[13] Farruggia P, DiMarco F, Dufour C. Pearson syndrome. Expert Rev. Hematol.2018;11:239-246. DOI: 10.1080/17474086.2018.1426454

[14] Maceluch JA, Niedziela M. The clinical diagnosis and molecular genetics of kearns-sayre syndrome: a complex mitochondrial encephalomyopathy. Pediatr Endocrinol Rev. 2006;4(2):117-137

[15] Van Goethem G, Martin JJ, Van Broeckhoven C. Progressive external ophthalmoplegia characterized by multiple deletions of mitochondrial DNA: unraveling the pathogenesis of human mitochondrial DNA instability and the initiation of a genetic classification. Neuromolecular Med. 2003;3(3):129-146. DOI: 10.1385/NMM:3:3:129

[16] Tatuch Y, Christodoulou J, Feigenbaum A, Clarke JT, Wherret J, Smith C, Rudd N, Petrova-Benedict R,

Robinson BH. HeteroplasmicmtDNA mutation (T----G) at 8993 can cause Leigh disease when the percentage of abnormal mtDNA is high. Am J Hum Genet. 1992;50(4):852-858

[17] Rahman S, Poulton J. Diagnosis of mitochondrial DNA depletion syndromes. Arch Dis Child. 2009;94(1):3-5. DOI: 10.1136/adc.2008.147983

[18] Lorenzoni PJ, Werneck LC, Kay CS, Silvado CE, Scola RH. When should MELAS (Mitochondrial myopathy, Encephalopathy, Lactic Acidosis, and Stroke-like episodes) be the diagnosis? ArqNeuropsiquiatr. 2015;73(11):959-967. DOI: 10.1590/0004-282X20150154

[19] Wang YX, Le WD. Progress in Diagnosing Mitochondrial Myopathy, Encephalopathy, Lactic Acidosis, and Stroke-like Episodes. Chin Med J (Engl). 2015;128(13):1820-1825. DOI: 10.4103/0366-6999.159360

[20] Goto Y, Nonaka I, Horai S. A mutation in the tRNA(Leu)(UUR) gene associated with the MELAS subgroup of mitochondrial encephalomyopathies. Nature. 1990;348(6302):651-653. DOI: 10.1038/348651a0

[21] Taylor RW, Chinnery PF, Haldane F, Morris AA, Bindoff LA, Wilson J, Turnbull DM. MELAS associated with a mutation in the valine transfer RNA gene of mitochondrial DNA. Ann Neurol. 1996;40(3):459-462. DOI: 10.1002/ana.410400318

[22] Manfredi G, Schon EA, Moraes CT, Bonilla E, Berry GT, Sladky JT, DiMauro S. A new mutation associated with MELAS is located in a mitochondrial DNA polypeptide-coding gene. NeuromusculDisord. 1995;5(5):391-398. DOI: 10.1016/0960-8966(94)00079-o

[23] Santorelli FM, Tanji K, Kulikova R, Shanske S, Vilarinho L, Hays AP, DiMauro S. Identification of a novel mutation in the mtDNA ND5 gene associated with MELAS. BiochemBiophys Res Commun. 1997;238(2):326-328. DOI: 10.1006/bbrc.1997.7167

[24] Shanske S, Coku J, Lu J, Ganesh J, Krishna S, Tanji K, Bonilla E, Naini AB, Hirano M, DiMauro S. The G13513A mutation in the ND5 gene of mitochondrial DNA as a common cause of MELAS or Leigh syndrome: evidence from 12 cases. Arch Neurol. 2008;65(3):368-372. DOI: 10.1001/archneurol.2007.67

[25] Corona P, Antozzi C, Carrara F, D'Incerti L, Lamantea E, Tiranti V, Zeviani M. A novel mtDNA mutation in the ND5 subunit of complex I in two MELAS patients. Ann Neurol. 200;49(1):106-110. DOI: 10.1002/1531-8249(200101)49:1<106::aid-ana16>3.0.co;2-t

[26] Liolitsa D, Rahman S, Benton S, Carr LJ, Hanna MG. Is the mitochondrial complex I ND5 gene a hot-spot for MELAS causing mutations? Ann Neurol. 2003;53(1):128-132. DOI: 10.1002/ana.10435

[27] Mancuso M, Petrozzi L, Filosto M, Nesti C, Rocchi A, Choub A, Pistolesi S, Massetani R, Fontanini G, Siciliano G. MERRF syndrome without ragged-red fibers: the need for molecular diagnosis. BiochemBiophys Res Commun. 2007 Mar;354(4):1058-1060. DOI: 10.1016/j.bbrc.2007.01.099

[28] Liu K, Zhao H, Ji K, Yan C. MERRF/MELAS overlap syndrome due to the m.3291T>C mutation. Metab Brain Dis. 2014;29(1):139-144. DOI: 10.1007/s11011-013-9464-5

[29] Hahn A, Schänzer A, Neubauer BA, Gizewski E, Ahting U,

Rolinski B. MERRF-like phenotype associated with a rare mitochondrial tRNAIle mutation (m.4284 G>A). Neuropediatrics. 2011;42(4):148-151. DOI: 10.1055/s-0031-1283167

[30] Cwerman-Thibault H, Augustin S, Ellouze S, Sahel JA, Corral-Debrinski M. Gene therapy for mitochondrial diseases: Leber Hereditary Optic Neuropathy as the first candidate for a clinical trial. C R Biol. 2014;337(3):193-206. DOI: 10.1016/j.crvi.2013.11.011

[31] Boggan RM, Lim A, Taylor RW, McFarland R, Pickett SJ. Resolving complexity in mitochondrial disease: Towards precision medicine. Mol Genet Metab. 2019;128(1-2):19-29. DOI: 10.1016/j.ymgme.2019.09.003

[32] Schon EA. Mitochondrial genetics and disease. Trends in Biochemical Sciences. 2000; 25(11):555-560. DOI: 10.1016/S0968-0004(00)01688-1

[33] Stenton SL, Prokisch H. Genetics of mitochondrial diseases: Identifying mutations to help diagnosis. EBioMedicine. 2020;56:102784. DOI: 10.1016/j.ebiom.2020.102784

[34] Tuppen HA, Blakely EL, Turnbull DM, Taylor RW. Mitochondrial DNA mutations and human disease. BiochimBiophys Acta. 2010;1797(2):113-128. DOI: 10.1016/j.bbabio.2009.09.005

[35] Rossignol R, Faustin B, Rocher C, Malgat M, Mazat JP, Letellier T. Mitochondrial threshold effects. Biochem J. 2003;370(Pt 3):751-762. DOI: 10.1042/BJ20021594

[36] Ghosh SS, Fahy E, Bodis-Wollner I, Sherman J, Howell N. Longitudinal study of a heteroplasmic 3460 Leber hereditary optic neuropathy family by multiplexed primer-extension analysis and nucleotide sequencing. Am J Hum Genet. 1996;58(2):325-334

[37] Larsson NG, Tulinius MH, Holme E, Oldfors A, Andersen O, Wahlström J, Aasly J. Segregation and manifestations of the mtDNA tRNA(Lys) A-->G(8344) mutation of myoclonus epilepsy and ragged-red fibers (MERRF) syndrome. Am J Hum Genet. 1992;51(6):1201-1212

[38] Marlow FL. Mitochondrial matters: Mitochondrial bottlenecks, self-assembling structures, and entrapment in the female germline. Stem Cell Res. 2017;21:178-186. DOI: 10.1016/j.scr.2017.03.004

[39] Yasuzaki Y, Yamada Y, Kanefuji T, Harashima H. Localization of exogenous DNA to mitochondria in skeletal muscle following hydrodynamic limb vein injection. J Control Release. 2013;172(3):805-811. DOI: 10.1016/j.jconrel.2013.09.029

[40] Bonnefoy N, Fox TD. Directed alteration of *Saccharomyces cerevisiae* mitochondrial DNA by biolistic transformation and homologous recombination. Methods Mol Biol. 2007;372:153-166. DOI: 10.1007/978-1-59745-365-3_11

[41] Cardoso AM, Morais CM, Cruz AR, Cardoso AL, Silva SG, do Vale ML, Marques EF, Pedroso de Lima MC, Jurado AS. Gemini surfactants mediate efficient mitochondrial gene delivery and expression. Mol Pharm. 2015;12(3):716-730. DOI: 10.1021/mp5005349

[42] Santos J, Sousa F, Queiroz J, Costa D. Rhodamine based plasmid DNA nanoparticles for mitochondrial gene therapy. Colloids Surf B Biointerfaces. 2014;121:129-140. DOI: 10.1016/j.colsurfb.2014.06.003

[43] D'Souza GG, Rammohan R, Cheng SM, Torchilin VP, Weissig V. DQAsome-mediated delivery of plasmid DNA toward mitochondria in living cells. J Control Release. 2003;92(1-2):189-197. DOI: 10.1016/s0168-3659(03)00297-9

[44] Yamada Y, Fukuda Y, Harashima H. An analysis of membrane fusion between mitochondrial double membranes and MITO-Porter, mitochondrial fusogenic vesicles. Mitochondrion. 2015;24:50-55. DOI: 10.1016/j.mito.2015.07.003

[45] Yamada Y, Ishikawa T, Harashima H. Validation of the use of an artificial mitochondrial reporter DNA vector containing a Cytomegalovirus promoter for mitochondrial transgene expression. Biomaterials. 2017;136:56-66. DOI: 10.1016/j.biomaterials.2017.05.016

[46] Chinnery PF, Taylor RW, Diekert K, Lill R, Turnbull DM, Lightowlers RN. Peptide nucleic acid delivery to human mitochondria. Gene Ther. 1999;6(12):1919-1928. DOI: 10.1038/sj.gt.3301061

[47] Flierl A, Jackson C, Cottrell B, Murdock D, Seibel P, Wallace DC. Targeted delivery of DNA to the mitochondrial compartment via import sequence-conjugated peptide nucleic acid. Mol Ther. 2003;7(4):550-557. DOI: 10.1016/s1525-0016(03)00037-6

[48] Yu H, Koilkonda RD, Chou TH, Porciatti V, Ozdemir SS, Chiodo V, Boye SL, Boye SE, Hauswirth WW, Lewin AS, Guy J. Gene delivery to mitochondria by targeting modified adenoassociated virus suppresses Leber's hereditary optic neuropathy in a mouse model. Proc Natl Acad Sci U S A. 2012;109(20):E1238-247. DOI: 10.1073/pnas.1119577109

[49] Yu H, Mehta A, Wang G, Hauswirth WW, Chiodo V, Boye SL, Guy J. Next-generation sequencing of mitochondrial targeted AAV transfer of human ND4 in mice. Mol Vis. 2013;19:1482-91

[50] Jang YH, Lim KI. Recent Advances in Mitochondria-Targeted Gene Delivery. Molecules. 2018;23(9):2316. DOI: 10.3390/molecules23092316

[51] Bacman SR, Gammage PA, Minczuk M, Moraes CT. Chapter 19 – Manipulation of mitochondrial genes and mtDNAheteroplasmy. Methods in Cell Biology. Academic Press. 2020;155:441-487. DOI: 10.1016/bs.mcb.2019.12.004

[52] Gammage PA, Rorbach J, Vincent AI, Rebar EJ, Minczuk M. Mitochondrially targeted ZFNs for selective degradation of pathogenic mitochondrial genomes bearing large-scale deletions or point mutations. EMBO Mol Med. 2014;6(4):458-466. DOI: 10.1002/emmm.201303672

[53] Gammage PA, Van Haute L, Minczuk M. Engineered mtZFNs for Manipulation of Human Mitochondrial DNA Heteroplasmy. Methods Mol Biol. 2016;1351:145-162. DOI: 10.1007/978-1-4939-3040-1_11

[54] Hashimoto M, Bacman SR, Peralta S, Falk MJ, Chomyn A, Chan DC, Williams SL, Moraes CT. MitoTALEN: A General Approach to Reduce Mutant mtDNA Loads and Restore Oxidative Phosphorylation Function in Mitochondrial Diseases. Mol Ther. 2015;23(10):1592-1599. DOI: 10.1038/mt.2015.126

[55] Gammage PA, Moraes CT, Minczuk M. Mitochondrial Genome Engineering: The Revolution May Not Be CRISPR-Ized. Trends Genet. 2018;34(2):101-110. DOI: 10.1016/j.tig.2017.11.001.

[56] Cerutti R, Pirinen E, Lamperti C, Marchet S, Sauve AA, Li W, Leoni V, Schon EA, Dantzer F, Auwerx J, Viscomi C, Zeviani M. NAD(+)-dependent activation of Sirt1 corrects the phenotype in a mouse model of mitochondrial disease. Cell Metab. 2014;19(6):1042-1049. DOI: 10.1016/j.cmet.2014.04.001

[57] Cantó C, Menzies KJ, Auwerx J. NAD(+) Metabolism and the Control of Energy Homeostasis: A Balancing Act between Mitochondria and the Nucleus. Cell Metab. 2015;22(1):31-53. DOI: 10.1016/j.cmet.2015.05.023

[58] Patgiri A, Skinner OS, Miyazaki Y, Schleifer G, Marutani E, Shah H, Sharma R, Goodman RP, To TL, Robert Bao X, Ichinose F, Zapol WM, Mootha VK. An engineered enzyme that targets circulating lactate to alleviate intracellular NADH:NAD+ imbalance. Nat Biotechnol. 2020;38(3):309-313. DOI: 10.1038/s41587-019-0377-7

[59] Tachibana M, Amato P, Sparman M, Woodward J, Sanchis DM, Ma H, Gutierrez NM, Tippner-Hedges R, Kang E, Lee HS, Ramsey C, Masterson K, Battaglia D, Lee D, Wu D, Jensen J, Patton P, Gokhale S, Stouffer R, Mitalipov S. Towards germline gene therapy of inherited mitochondrial diseases. Nature. 2013;493(7434):627-631. DOI: 10.1038/nature11647

[60] Hyslop LA, Blakeley P, Craven L, Richardson J, Fogarty NM, Fragouli E, Lamb M, Wamaitha SE, Prathalingam N, Zhang Q, O'Keefe H, Takeda Y, Arizzi L, Alfarawati S, Tuppen HA, Irving L, Kalleas D, Choudhary M, Wells D, Murdoch AP, Turnbull DM, Niakan KK, Herbert M. Towards clinical application of pronuclear transfer to prevent mitochondrial DNA disease. Nature. 2016;534(7607):383-386. DOI: 10.1038/nature18303

[61] Russell OM, Gorman GS, Lightowlers RN, Turnbull DM. Mitochondrial Diseases: Hope for the Future. Cell. 2020;181(1):168-188. DOI: 10.1016/j.cell.2020.02.051

Section 2

Model Organisms and Mutagenesis

Chapter 5

Mouse Models to Understand Mutagenic Outcomes and Illegitimate Repair of DNA Damage

Kiran Lalwani, Caroline French and Christine Richardson

Abstract

Maintenance of genome integrity is critical to prevent cell death or disease. Illegitimate repair of chromosomal DNA breaks can lead to mutations and genome rearrangements which are a well-known hallmark of multiple cancers and disorders. Endogenous causes of DNA double-strand breaks (DSBs) include reactive oxygen species (ROS) and replication errors while exogenous causes of DNA breaks include ionizing radiation, UV radiation, alkylating agents, and inhibitors of topoisomerase II (Top2). Recent evidence suggests that a growing list of environmental agents or toxins and natural dietary compounds also cause DNA breaks. Understanding the consequences of exposure to a broad spectrum of DSB-inducing agents has significant implications for understanding mutagenicity, genome stability and human health. This chapter will review *in vivo* mouse models designed to measure DNA damage and mutagenicity, and illegitimate repair of DNA DSBs caused by exposure to environmental agents.

Keywords: mutagenicity, double-strand breaks, illegitimate repair, genome rearrangement, transgenic mouse model, genome instability

1. Introduction

The faithful repair of DNA lesions is central to the maintenance of genomic integrity [1]. Illegitimate repair of chromosomal DNA breaks can lead to mutations and genome rearrangements which are a well-known hallmark of multiple cancers, aging, and disease [2, 3]. DSBs can occur in a programmed manner during a metabolic process such as DNA replication, during meiosis, and the development of the immune system during V(D)J recombination and immunoglobulin class switch recombination [4] or endogenous agents such as ROS and replication errors [5]. DSBs also occur as a result of exposure to exogenous agents such as ionizing radiation, UV radiation, alkylating agents, topoisomerase inhibitors, and chemotherapeutic drugs [6–8]. Evidence shows that a growing list of natural compounds in the human diet or the environment also causes DNA breaks [9].

Mammalian cells have evolved sophisticated mechanisms to detect the damage via the DNA damage response (DDR) and signaling pathway which then activates repair pathways to maintain genome integrity [10]. Major mammalian processes to detect and repair DNA DSBs include homologous recombination (HR) and non-homologous end joining (NHEJ) (**Figure 1**). Both of these repair pathways are cell cycle-specific and differ based on their requirement for a donor DNA template with significant DNA sequence similarity. Studies suggest NHEJ is most prevalent in non-cycling somatic cells during the G1 stage, while HR is particularly active during the S, G2, and M stages due to its requirement for a homologous sequence as a donor template [11, 12]. In NHEJ the broken ends are processed and ligated together without

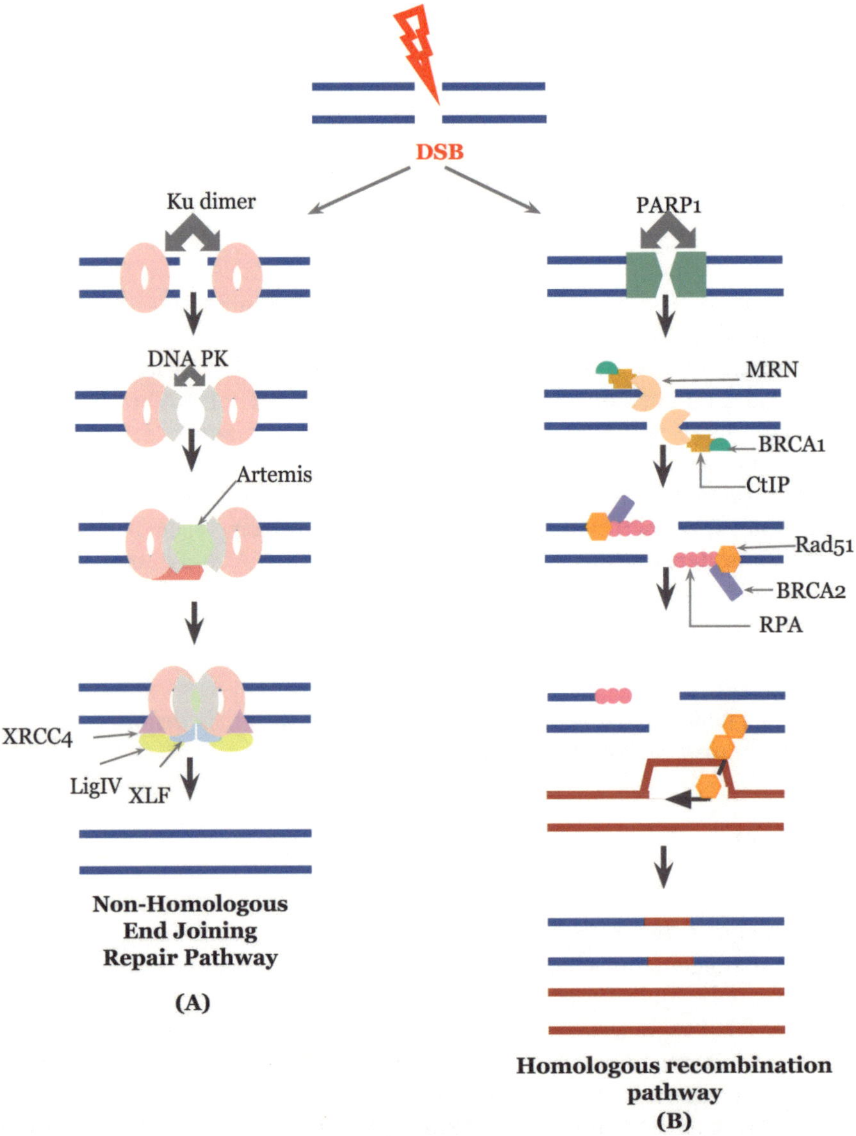

Figure 1.
The DNA double-strand breaks (DSB) are repaired by the two pathways; These are—(A) non-homologous end joining (C-NHEJ) which modifies the ends and allows ligation of the broken ends to repair the DSB; (B) homologous recombination (HR) that uses a homologous sequence from sister chromatid or homologous chromosome or a homologous sequence within the genome.

requiring homology. By contrast, HR uses an undamaged homologous sequence from a sister chromatid, allelic locus, or an ectopically located sequence from a heterologous chromosome as a template to initiate HR or break-induced replication repair at the broken site [13].

Laboratory mice (*Mus musculus*) have been key to most *in vivo* studies on DNA damage and mutagenicity or illegitimate repair that take into account the complex environment of the mammalian system including tissue architecture, cellular differentiation programs, chromatin landscape patterns, and aging [14–18]. Multiple *in vivo* models have been developed to examine the potential for the repair of DNA DSBs [19, 20]. Furthermore, specific cell types within tissues and organs encounter a diverse set of DNA damaging insults that produce distinct types of DNA damage. Individual cells differ in their capacity for sensing, responding, and repairing specific DNA lesions [17].

2. Induction and assessment of mutagenicity by endogenous sources

2.1 Programmed DNA DSBs

Endogenous DNA DSBs can occur as deliberate, cell-required mechanisms. DNA DSBs drive the non-sister chromatid HR events responsible for genetic diversity in meiotic cells [21]. These events can lead to rearrangements including deletions, tandem duplications, inversions, and translocation of chromosomes which are not always favorable for the cell [22]. Analogous to topoisomerase II (Top2), the Spo11 enzyme initiates DSBs during prophase I of meiosis. The locations Spo11-mediated DSBs are not random and are referred to as DNA hotspots expected to occur somewhere between 10,000 and 40,000 times within the mammalian genome [23]. These DSBs initiate meiotic HR via gene conversion and crossover events. Spo11$^{-/-}$ knockout mice have errors in normal meiotic chromosome synapsis formation [24]. PRDM9 methyltransferase and its associated binding specificity determine the DSB hotspot locations in mice by generating nucleosome-depleted regions, allowing for the programmed DSBs to occur via Spo11 cleavage [25].

2.2 Reactive oxygen species and replication stress

DNA DSBs can occur due to the accumulation of ROS-induced oxidative stress or as the result of replication or transcription stress. ROS are often linked to neurological diseases and cancer, although they result from endogenous cellular metabolism. Some examples of endogenous ROS include the superoxide radical anion ($O_2^{\cdot -}$), hydroxyl radical ($OH^{\cdot}$), peroxynitrite ($ONOO^-$), and hypochlorous acid (HOCl) [26]. ROS cause DNA damage through their ability to alter the overall reduction-oxidation (redox) cell conditions to cause oxidative stress. By changing redox conditions of the cell, important cellular processes including signal transduction and proliferation may not be able to occur. The failure of these processes can be lethal for the cell or promote mutagenesis through GC to TA changes [27]. Guanine lesions that lead to a miscoding error change the structural integrity of the DNA by weakening hydrogen bonding between bases [26]. These guanine mutations are associated with ROS-related oxidative stress and can promote cancer development [27]. 8-Oxo-7,8-dihydroguanine (8-oxoG) is a common output of guanine oxidation. It is an important compound because of its susceptibility to further oxidation and overall genotoxicity [28].

The base excision repair (BER) pathway is a mechanism deployed to resolve DNA lesions, as the presence of 8-oxoG, and has three major steps: (1) recognition of the lesion by DNA glycosylases, (2) base excision, (3) resynthesis and replacement of the removed base [29]. DNA glycosylases initiate BER through cleaving the *N*-glycosidic bond between the damaged base and sugar. DNA glycosylases can be either monofunctional or bi-functional whereas bi-functional DNA glycosylases include a β-elimination or β, δ-elimination step after *N*-glycosidic bond cleavage [30]. Defects in the BER pathway's mechanism can lead to the accumulation of BER intermediates, unrepaired lesions, point mutations, and DNA DSBs. DNA polymerase β (Pol β) is one of the most active DNA polymerases involved in BER. A single nucleotide polymorphism (SNP) on the gene coding for Pol β results in proline residue 242 becoming arginine (P242R). This mutation is suggested to cause chromosomal aberrations, and therefore, genome instability. P242R was associated with an increase in SSBs and DSBs compared to wild-type cells, and cellular transformation in mouse and human cells. An observed increase in cellular proliferation with the expression of the P242R suggested this mutation may induce a carcinogenic phenotype [31].

Replication stress is any event causing changes to the replication rate and can include halting replication. Unrepaired DNA lesions contribute to replication stress by acting as a physical block of the replication fork and its motion [32]. Single strand breaks (SSBs) generated by replication stress can further generate DSBs by nucleases, deamination, or spontaneous hydrolysis [22]. These DSBs, as well as meiotic-related DSBs, will use NHEJ or HR for repair. Errors in HR, which are less common than in NHEJ, can lead to mutagenesis and overall genome instability [33]. Phosphorylation of target proteins by ATM also triggers DDR. Chk2 has protein kinase activity allowing it to phosphorylate several effector proteins in the cell cycle checkpoint including p53 which can be modified by either ATM or Chk2 (or ATR or Chk1). ARF protein (p14) seems to stabilize TIP60 interactions with ATM for better activation and is associated with maintaining genome stability [2].

2.3 Spontaneous DNA breaks

A reporter fluorescent yellow direct repeat (FYDR) mouse model was developed to assess DSB-induced intra-chromosomal recombination events in multiple tissues including skin [34, 35]. In this model, spontaneous DSBs or DSBs induced by replication fork collapse can lead to unequal sister chromatid exchange between tandem truncated enhanced yellow fluorescent protein (EYFP) sequences resulting in gene conversion and expression of EYFP quantifiable by flow cytometry. This model showed the *in vivo* frequency of spontaneous intra-chromosomal HR in multiple tissues calculated at approximately 10^{-5} to 10^{-6} per base pair per cell division. A modification of the model using a direct repeat-GFP (RaDR-GFP) inserted in the Rosa*26* locus contains two truncated EGFP sequences in tandem [14, 34–36]. This model detected spontaneous and DNA damage agent-induced intra-chromosomal HR in most gastrointestinal organs and respiratory organs. Cell-type-specific immunohistochemistry staining of the lung [36] and pancreata [35] demonstrated cell-type and tissue-type specificity of intra-chromosomal HR recombinant populations. This model also demonstrated that older mice show an order of magnitude increase in the accumulation of recombinant cells.

3. Induction and assessment of mutagenicity by exogenous agents

Exposure of mice to nonspecific agents such as IR, Top2 inhibitors and chemotherapeutic drugs induce DSBs more broadly across the genome and in physiologically relevant contexts (**Figure 2**).

3.1 Ionizing and non-ionizing radiation

Ionizing radiations such as X-rays and gamma rays can cause direct damage by depositing energy or indirect damage by ionization of water molecules to produce free radicals that influence SSBs or DSBs [37–40]. The complexities of the damage vary according to the linear energy transfer of the radiation [37]. Alpha particles are high LET radiation and directly cause breaks [41] while non-ionizing radiations such as UVA and UVB create indirect DSBs and SSBs [7]. Several DSB repair pathway-specific proteins have been examined on bases of the IR sensitivity such as MRE1 resection protein [42], BRCA1 [43], Ku 70 [44], and Pol θ [45–47]. Exposure of mice to irradiation can cause a variety of DNA lesions including base damage, SSBs and DSBs. However, DSBs have been deduced to be amongst the toxic lesions and contribute to cell death [37]. Erroneous repair of the DSBs causes chromosomal aberrations and influences carcinogenesis [38].

The earliest methods for detection of DSBs induced by irradiation included physical separation of the broken DNA from undamaged DNA by pulse-field gel electrophoresis and comet assays [47, 48]. However, these methods were not efficient for mouse studies because of their low reproducibility and limited approximation of DSB levels [50]. More recently, micronuclei scoring is more commonly used as these cytogenetic biomarkers are easily detectable through microscopy. Micronuclei are cytoplasmic chromatin masses resulting from damaging agents such as IR [49, 50]. Another prominent and widely used method for the detection of DSBs include the identification of DSB downstream biomarkers such as γH2AX that binds to DNA at sites flanking DSBs [51, 52]. This protein is a variant of H2AX histone and forms a focus at the sites of DSBs which further signals DDR and repair response [50, 51]. The γH2AX foci can be analyzed by immunohistochemical staining and visualization under fluorescent or confocal microscopy.

To determine the repair pathway choice of DSB repair association of DSBs with proteins specific for one pathway or another is typically employed. For example, HR requires resection of the broken DNA ends from ssDNAs that are recognized and covered by replication protein A (RPA) which can be detected through immunofluorescence. To monitor the length and speed of resection per DNA molecule, BrdU antibody is used which binds to the ssDNA and forms fibers visible under a fluorescent microscope. To increase the resolution of DNA fibers, Single-Molecule Analysis of Resection Tracks (SMART) can be used [53, 54].

3.2 Radiomimetic drugs

Commonly used chemotherapeutic drugs are categorized into 5 different types based upon their chemical composition and mode of action. Widely used anti-cancer drugs for DNA damage include alkylating agents such as temozolomide (TMZ) melphalan, and cyclophosphamide [55, 56]. These agents act by attaching the alkyl groups onto the DNA and interfering with the cell cycle and transcription process.

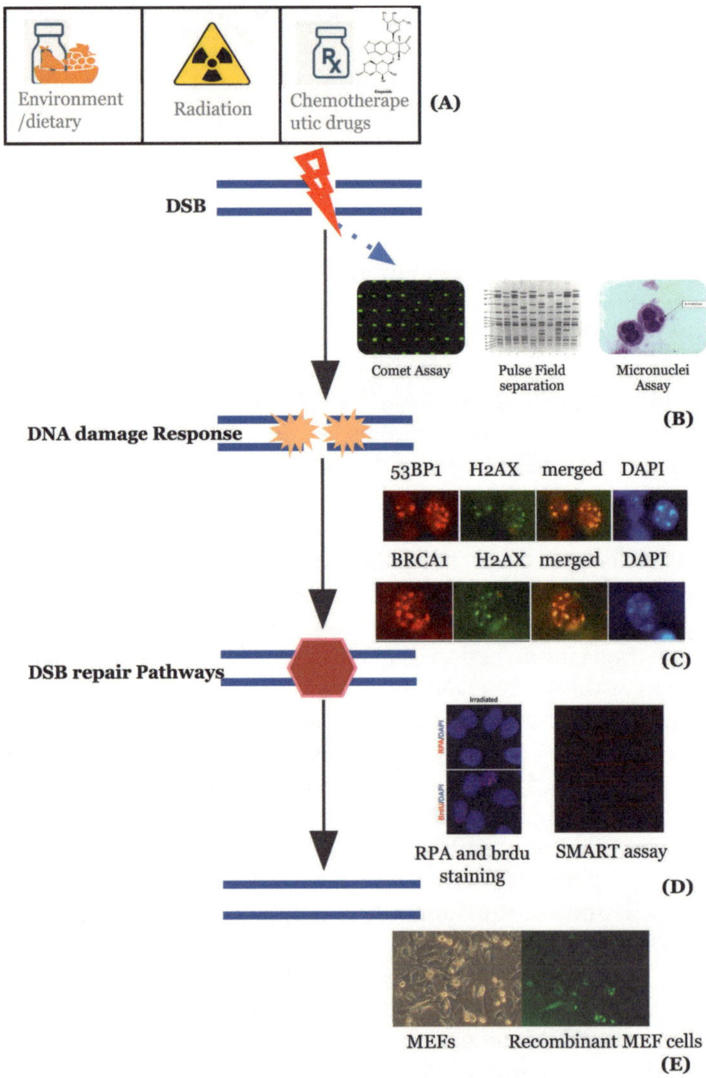

Figure 2.
Exogenous exposure DNA double strand break induction, damage response pathway and repair. (A) The schematic figure shows induction of DNA damage via chemotherapeutics, radiation and environmental compounds. (B) The preliminary assessment of the DSB can be done by techniques such as comet assay, pulse electrophoresis and micronuclei staining. (C) Detection DNA damage response proteins such gamma H2AX, 53BP1 and BRCA1 foci using immunofluorescence staining. (D) Hr specific techniques such as SMART assay and brdu staining. (E) To determine repair frequencies several reporters are developed. For example, GFP recombinant cells shown in bottom right.

They can also cross-link two double-strand DNA molecules creating inter-strand cross-links (ICLs). ICLs are dangerous lesions if not repaired. Alkylating agents can also add mismatched nucleotides which can cause genome instability [56]. Studies targeting DDR and DSB repair proteins that can alter the sensitivity of chemotherapeutic drugs are used for cancer treatment modalities. Recent research proposed that deficiency of the NHEJ protein DNA ligase4 significantly enhanced the sensitivity of cells to TMZ [57]. Mouse embryonic fibroblasts (MEFs) of DNA ligase 4 knockout mice treated with a D50 dose of TMZ have higher numbers γH2AX foci and significantly reduced cell survival when compared to wild-type suggesting that Ligase4 protects the cells against lesions from TMZ [57].

ICL-inducing agents, such as mitomycin C (MMC), nitrogen mustards, and platinum can create cross-links that hinder DNA replication, thus preferentially targeting highly proliferative cells. Thus, these agents are widely used in the treatment of cancers and several skin conditions [55, 58]. The repair of ICLs involves both translesion break repair and HR proteins, and mutation of HR genes leads to sensitivity to ICL agents [59, 60]. Brca1 mutant mice ear fibroblasts and MEFs treated with MMC showed significantly reduced HR frequency and increased sensitivity to MMC. Interestingly, ATM mutant mice did not have a significant change in HR frequency even with higher MMC doses suggesting that ATM is dispensable for HR [59].

Molecular studies indicate the necessity of Top2 in the maintenance of genome integrity. The ability to halt Top2 function and generate enzyme-mediated DNA damage is a key reason why it is used in secondary cancer chemotherapy such as therapy-related acute myeloid leukemia (t-AML) [61, 62]. Top2 enzyme acts by catalyzing the interconversion of topological DNA isomers through the generation of a transient DSB on one DNA helix ("gate" strand) while remaining covalently linked to the 5′ end of the DNA, followed by passage of a second DNA helix ("transfer" strand) through the DSB, and then religation of the DSB [63]. Mammals have two isoforms of Top2—α and β [61]. Chemotherapeutic drugs doxorubicin and etoposide inhibit the catalytic activity of Top2 after generating the DSB resulting in high levels of trapped Top2:DNA complexes and unrepaired DSBs [9, 61]. Such agents are also referred to as Top2 "poisons" [61]. A novel insight into secondary malignancies induced by these Top2 targeting drugs has come from studies using a transgenic mouse model with a skin-specific ablation of Top2β [63]. These skin-specific *top2*β-knockout mice were exposed to etoposide to evaluate the role of the two isozymes of DNA, Top2α and Top2β. The results demonstrated that in the absence of Top2β, there was a reduction in NHEJ induced by etoposide, suggesting a potential role of NHEJ repair in promoting the malignancies created by improper repair of these lesions [64, 65].

3.3 Pollutants and environmental compounds

Chemical compounds including air and water pollutants, pesticides and some dietary compounds are genotoxic and linked to carcinogenesis. Air pollutants such as benzene and sulfur oxide are released by the combustion of fossil fuels are often linked with leukemias [65, 66]. An *in vivo* study demonstrated how benzoquinone (BQ) environmental agent-induced recombination in fetal hematopoietic cells in pKZ1 transgenic mice [67]. BQ potentially induced ROS measured by a significant increase in the ROS product 8-OH-2′-dG. This was followed by DSB induction that was detected by a significant increase in γH2AX foci in the BQ treated cells. The widely used pesticide endosulfan is speculated to cause chromosomal abnormalities in humans [68, 69]. Adult wild-type BALB/c mice fed endosulfan and analyzed for DSBs and ROS-mediated damage showed an increase in γH2AX foci and a significant increase in the levels of the NHEJ-associated protein 53BP1 in lungs and testes. Furthermore, elevations of several other proteins involved in the alternative end joining (Alt-EJ) pathway were evaluated by Western blot. This study provided compelling insight on the mechanism of action of endosulfan pesticide [69].

Bisphenol A (BPA) is a hormonally active environmental xenoestrogen widely found in food products. It is an epigenetic toxicant that can alter the DNA by the generation of ROS [70]. Bioflavonoids are polyphenolic compounds found in various dietary products such as soy, coffee, fruits, and vegetables [71]. These compounds have been characterized to be mechanistically and biochemically similar to the Top2 inhibitor and chemotherapeutic drug etoposide [72, 73]. In addition, bioflavonoids have been shown to cross the placental barrier and can induce *MLL* breakpoint cluster region cleavage suggesting an association with the initiation of infant leukemia [74]. A study reported prenatal exposure to flavonoids genistein or quercetin can increase the risk for leukemia onset, as assessed by the frequency of *MLL* translocations in an ATM mutant mouse model prone to develop cancer [75]. Prenatally exposed fetuses were examined at gestation day 14.5 by inverse-PCR to detect *MLL* translocations and their frequency in the fetal liver. Additionally, mice prenatally exposed to flavonoids genistein or quercetin were euthanized at 12-weeks and inverse PCR was performed to determine the presence of *MLL* translocations. These prenatally exposed mice developed leukemia albeit at later ages [75]. These results are further supported by an embryonic stem cell GFP-NHEJ model to identify chromosomal translocations between *MLL* and *AF9* breakpoint cluster regions analogous to those observed in infant leukemia [76]. Upon damage induced by etoposide or a large panel of flavonoids, DSBs in the two loci and repair by NHEJ produced a chromosomal translocation resulting in a functional full-length GFP at least partly dependent on Top2 [76, 77]. Another study examined epigenetic effects of genistein on hematopoiesis in mice; mice prenatally exposed to genistein showed the significant increase in erythropoiesis. Furthermore, transcriptional microarray analysis suggested that genistein exposure was associated with hypermethylation of certain repetitive elements which coincided with a significant down-regulation of genes involved in hematopoiesis in bone marrow cells and estrogen-responsive genes of genistein-exposed mice [78].

Another reporter system assesses mutagenic events through the *Escherichia coli*-derived LacZ gene, which codes for the production of β-galactosidase. β-Galactosidase cleaves lactose forming galactose and glucose, but is receptive to substrate 4-bromo-5-chloro-3-indolyl β-D-galactopyraniside (X-Gal) and produces blue precipitate when bound to β-galactosidase. The blue precipitate is observable through light microscopy [79]. Shuttle vectors carrying the bacterial reporter gene include micro-injection of bacteriophages and electroporation of plasmids for the development of transgenic mice for mutagenetic assay. Transgenic LacZ$^+$ mice have been dosed with different mutagenic chemical compounds, like ethyl nitrosourea, chlorambucil, and benzo[α]pyrene, to observe changes in the production of X-Gal's blue precipitate as an indicator of mutagenicity [80]. The Mutamouse and Big Blue transgenic mouse models were developed via bacteriophages. Mutamouse utilizes bacteriophage λ DNA (λ gt10) as a vector for LacZ insertion at an *Eco*RI restriction site. Excision of the LacZ gene for analysis and a positive agar selection system is used with scoring of the clear plaques to identify mutants. Big Blue also has a λ bacteriophage shuttle vector for LacZ, but a non-selectable color screening assay to provide a ratio of blue plaques to white plaques and consequently a mutation frequency [81]. In the 35.5 transgenic mouse system, the LacZ transgene concameter is in a particularly unstable chromosomal region near the pseudo-autosomal region on the X-chromosome resulting in an increased potential for germinal and somatic mutations [80].

4. Induction and assessment of mutagenicity by site-directed cleavage

Nonspecific DNA damaging agents including chemotherapeutic drugs, environmental agents and radiation provide a global understanding of cell function during the response to DNA damage and DSBs. Molecular analysis of specific repair is difficult as spontaneously occurring DNA breaks occur in unknown locations. Off-target effects on the genome can be limited by using tools such as endonucleases and retroviruses. In addition to site-specific damage induced by specific endonucleases, a defective selectable marker or a defective fluorescent protein such as green fluorescent protein (GFP) can be added to develop a reporter system [82]. The endonuclease induces DSBs, and repair can result in a fluorescent or selectable active marker that was previously defective (**Figure 3**).

4.1 Recombinase cleavage and repair reporters

Development of conditional and inducible *in vivo* reporter assays allows for manipulation of gene expression, and molecular identification of deletion or addition of DNA sequence at specific loci. Generally, a DNA recombinase enzyme is involved in the development of conditional reporter systems. Recombinase enzymes such as Cre and FRT catalyze a concerted recombination reaction between two target sequences (loxP for Cre and FRT for FLP). Depending on the relative orientation of the target sites, catalysis results in the excision of the DNA gene sequences between the target sequences [83, 84]. A conditional Nbs1 null mouse MEF system developed with cre-lox recombinase provided insight regarding the role of the MRE11, RAD50 and NBS1 (MRN) complex with other repair proteins in DSB processing and HR. Nbs1 null MEFs treated with MMC or IR followed by Western blotting and immunohistochemistry of Brca1 and Rad51 indicated that loss of Nbs1 affected single-strand annealing via Rad51 suggesting its role in promoting HR. In support of this, PCR and Southern blotting suggested that loss of Nbs1 in an embryonic stem cell line promoted NHEJ repair [85].

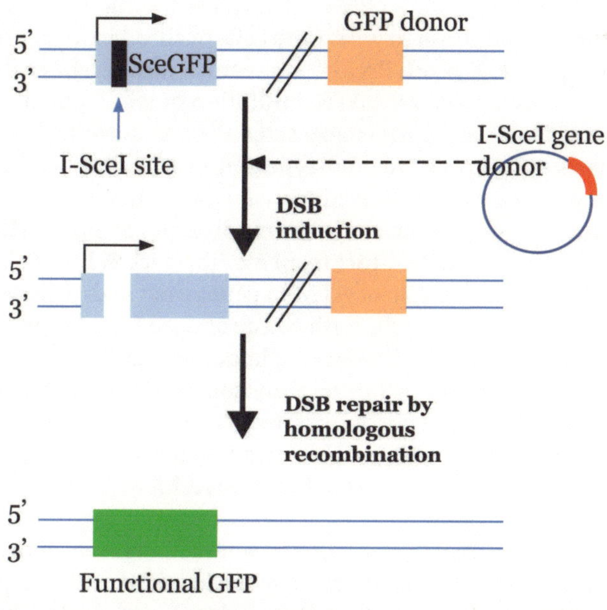

Figure 3.
Schematic of a GFP reporter system. This cassette consists of a ISceI-GFP is a modified GFP gene, which contains an 18 bp long ISceI recognition site and in-frame termination codons and a downstream a GFP donor fragment. Addition of an ISceI gene donor to this system induces DNA DSB at the ISceI site. Homologous recombination by gene conversion results in a functional GFP gene.

4.2 Endonuclease cleavage and repair reporters

Restriction enzymes can induce site-specific DSBs with their sequence specificity to target DNA. Intron specific encoded endonuclease 1 (IsceI) derived from *Saccharomyces cerevisiae* is one of the first endonucleases used for the study of HR in mammalian cells and, subsequently, *in vivo* [82, 86].

The G2S mouse model was developed to determine the potential for DSB-induced inter-chromosomal HR repair *in vivo* [84]. This G2S mouse model was genetically engineered to contain three distinct transgenes—two non-functional green fluorescent protein (GFP) reporter transgenes and a bi-cistronic doxycycline (Dox)-inducible IsceI transgene. Each GFP reporter construct contains an IsceI recognition site that renders it non-functional and provides for the induction of specific DSBs. Repair of the IsceI-induced DSBs by inter-chromosomal HR generates a functional GFP gene. While no GFP+ cells were detected without Dox ($<1 \times 10^{-8}$), following the addition of Dox to mouse chow or drinking water, fluorescent GFP+ cells were detected in a large spectrum of tissue types and hematopoietic progenitor cell populations visualized by fluorescent microscopy and quantitated by flow cytometry. Similar to results with RaDR mice and intra-chromosomal HR, aged G2S mice showed reduced numbers of inter-chromosomal HR cell populations [87].

Another study examined the genetic interactions between ATM, BRCA1, and 53BP1 in mice using a hypomorphic mutant, $Brca1^{S1598F}$ ($Brca1^{SF}$) [88]. To study the role of these proteins in intra-chromosomal HR, primary fibroblasts from $Brca1^{SF/SF}$ mice and $Atm^{-/-}$ mice were integrated with a direct repeat GFP (DR-GFP) reporter and a Dox-inducible IsceI endonuclease. The DR-GFP contains a full-length nonfunctional GFP gene containing an IsceI endonuclease site followed by a downstream GFP homologous donor sequence; DSBs induced by IsceI cleavage can promote intra-chromosomal HR repair to result in GFP+ cells. While spontaneous GFP+ cells were minimal (<0.01%), Dox addition to wild-type cells resulted in detection of GFP+ cells indicating HR repair (3–4%). Both $Brca1^{SF}$ and $Atm^{-/-}$ models showed a 3- and 2-fold reduction in GFP+ cells, respectively. ATM inhibition in wild-type cells only reduced HR by 1.6-fold, while ATM inhibitor exacerbated the generation of GFP+ cells in $Brca1^{SF/SF}$ fibroblasts as compared to wild-type and $Atm^{-/-}$ fibroblasts. PCR-based assay with the DR-GFP reporter was used to quantify the SSA pathway which suggested significant reduction. Interaction of Atm, Brca and 53 bp1 in HR, was demonstrated by the appearance of RAD51 foci from ear fibroblasts. Examination of triple mutants indicated the plausible role of ATM in generating end-resected intermediates for RAD51 filament formation in cells with compromised BRCA1 and 53BP [88].

A recent age-dependent study developed a knock-in R26BHEJ model to determine the efficiency of frequency of intrachromosomal NHEJ for repair. R26BNHEJ knock-in is a GFP-based NHEJ reporter inserted into the ROSA26A locus. The DSBs are created using IsceI and repair by NHEJ was analyzed in several tissues using flow cytometry. This model demonstrated that there was a 1.8 to 3.8-fold decline of NHEJ efficiency with increased age [89].

In the past two decades, new approaches of gene editing have enormously expanded mutagenesis studies. Use of artificial nuclease like zinc-finger (ZFN), transcription activator-like effector (TALEN) nuclease, and the latest clustered regularly interspaced short palindromic repeat (CRISPR)/associated (Cas9) system has enhanced precision of gene editing [90, 91]. ZFN and TALEN nucleases consist of sequence-specific DNA-binding domains that are fused to a nonspecific DNA cleavage module such as FokI endonuclease. These systems readily search for sequence homology and the endonuclease cleaves at the recognition site, removing the target gene. Several development studies use ZFN and TALEN for gene editing [90]. A powerful approach for gene alteration is the CRISPR-Cas9 system. This system was initially observed in bacteria as an immune response against viruses. It consists of a single-guide RNA (sgRNA), that targets a palindromic region in the specific location of the genome, which is recognized by Cas9 nuclease generating a DNA DSB that subsequently activates the cellular DNA repair machinery. HR or NHEJ repair would result in alteration of the target gene by indel mutations [92, 93].

5. Induction and assessment of mutagenicity *in utero*

In utero studies can provide valuable insight into the physiological processes that make mammalian models unique. Although, the single-cell *Saccharomyces cerevisiae* has a large number of genes with homologs in mammals that are involved in DNA damage, signaling and repair [94], it is important to consider the mouse model's advantage to understanding DNA damage and repair in multiple organ systems that a single-cell model cannot provide. Oogenesis, embryogenesis, and spermatogenesis are processes that give valuable insight to mutagenicity because of their roles in development and meiotic recombination and their potential to lead to trans-generational mutational consequences.

5.1 Gametocyte-based assays

Understanding the mammalian recombination pathway is useful for developing mouse models that can be used to appropriately study meiotic recombination stress and DSB repair. Because knockout of MRN complex components causes embryonic lethality, conditional disruption of NBS1 has been utilized in germ cells to assess how the MRN complex is functioning during meiotic DSB repair in mice [95]. A germ cell-specific transgenic mouse model inactivates targeted gene expression utilizing *Vasa-cre* [95, 96]. In *Nbs1*$^{flox/-}$*;Vasa-Cre (Nbs1 vKO)* transgenic mice, NSB1 was conditionally knocked out preceding the time in meiotic development when Spo11-mediates DSBs. In this system, male mice were infertile. Zhang *et al.* observed improper chromosome synapsis using SYCP3 and γH2AX immunostaining of spermatocytes. Immunostaining also showed nuclear localization of MRE11 in the spermatocytes was disrupted by the depleted NBS1. Development of the Nbs1 vKO transgenic mouse model allowed for the assay of NBS1 as an indicator of MRN function, and in turn, meiotic recombination stress [95].

5.2 Applications

As modern healthcare concerns center around fetal development, mouse models can be used to understand how meiotic recombination is affected by compounds in our environment. Oogenesis is particularly important because the events of meiotic prophase I are highly influential on fetal survival. An *in utero* model has been used to assess fetal exposure to supplemented estrogen and how meiotic prophase I progression is altered in response. 17-ß-estradiol (E_2) was administered to pregnant mice. The meiotic outcomes were analyzed through γH2AX staining and examination by super-resolution structured illumination microscope where γH2AX presence would signify whether meiotic recombination occurred via the initiation of a DSB.

Quantifying γH2AX *in utero* is a valuable tool for assessing meiotic mutagenicity and then later influences fetal development and success [97].

In utero exposure to other environmental agents that cause DNA damage can be valuable for understanding carcinogenesis. The absence of the P53 tumor-suppressor gene is linked to spontaneous tumorigenesis [27, 98]. P53 knockout mice can be used as a model for assessing tumor development when exposed to cancer-causing agents. An *in utero* study evaluated the effects of high-dose vitamin E, hypothesized to have antioxidative properties, on tumorigenesis. Pregnant P53 knockout mice were fed high-dose vitamin E until gestation day 13 or gestation day 19. The addition of vitamin E altered the redox state of the *in utero* environment. Furthermore, the oxidative stress on the ROS-dependent embryonic and fetal pathways was evaluated. DNA isolation was performed for the fetal and embryonic tissues and high-performance liquid chromatography was used to quantify the formation of 8-oxo-dG which would be used as an oxidation marker. Vitamin E dosing was associated with an increase in tumorigenesis in the p53 knockout mice; however, further studies are needed to explore the relationship between vitamin E and the tumorigenesis pathway [27]. Assessing vitamins sold commercially is valuable to improving our understanding of what supplements are safe during pregnancy and how ROS may influence *in utero* cancer development.

Oxidative stress has important connections to ovarian aging because these ROS lesions in ovarian follicles increase with age. Oocytes remain dormant in the diplotene stage until they are released for fertilization providing time for ROS-induced oxidative damage lesions to accumulate, and an increase of these lesions in ovarian follicles with age [99]. Pol *β* and BER, a pathway for repairing DNA lesions caused by ROS and oxidative damage, have been associated with the aging process. As rats age, Pol *β* levels decline, and BER becomes less efficient [100]. Injection of small interfering RNA (siRNA) targeting Pol *β* into young murine oocytes resulted in decreased numbers of normal oocytes, reduced oocyte survival, and an increase in detectable 8-oxoG levels, as compared to controls. In a complementary study, injection of Pol *β* complementary DNA (cDNA) into aged murine oocytes resulted in overexpression of Pol *β*, increased oocyte survival, and a decrease in detectable 8-oxoG levels, as compared to controls. These studies suggest that Pol *β* function is important for oocyte survival and aging. There is a potential to apply the overexpression of Pol *β* in clinical settings to improve oocyte survival and potentially slow the damaging effects of DNA lesions on aging oocytes. This is a potentially important finding for improving fertility and pregnancy outcomes as aging signs of progress [99].

6. Conclusion

Genomic instability plays a prominent role in the initiation of pathologies such as aging, immunodeficiencies and carcinogenesis. To combat the lethal effect of DNA damage and strand breaks, cells have evolved multiple, often overlapping DNA repair pathways efficiently and accurately repair DNA. Induction and assessment of genotoxicant DNA damage are particularly important *in vivo*. Further, these mouse models to assess DNA damage and repair can be combined with traditional mouse genetics to determine the impact of genetic modifications or polymorphisms with a focus on molecular analysis of DNA damage repair. As the number of designed and widely used synthetic environmental agents increases, understanding their impact on DNA integrity and downstream potential to promote mutagenicity is increasingly significant.

Acknowledgements

CR was funded in part by NIH/NIGMS and a Faculty Research Grant (UNC Charlotte). KL was funded in part by Proposal Development Summer Fellowship (UNC Charlotte).

Conflict of interest

The authors indicate no conflict of interest.

Author details

Kiran Lalwani, Caroline French and Christine Richardson*
University of North Carolina at Charlotte, Charlotte, NC, USA

*Address all correspondence to: c.richardson@uncc.edu

References

[1] Lalwani K, Goodenow D, Richardson C. Eukaryotic Recombination: Initiation by Double-strand Breaks. In: Encyclopedia of Life Sciences. Hoboken, New Jersey: John Wiley & Sons, Ltd. 2020;**1**:69-76

[2] Ciccia A, Elledge SJ. The DNA damage response: Making it safe to play with knives. Molecular Cell. 2010;**40**(2):179

[3] Hoeijmakers JHJ. Molecular origins of cancer DNA damage, aging, and cancer. The New England Journal of Medicine. 2009;**361**:1475-1485

[4] Jung D, Alt FW. Unraveling V(D)J recombination: Insights into gene regulation. Cell. 2004;**116**(2):299-311

[5] Lindahl T, Barnes DE. Repair of endogenous DNA damage. Cold Spring Harbor Symposia on Quantitative Biology. 2000;**65**:127-133

[6] Wogan GN, Hecht SS, Felton JS, Conney AH, Loeb LA. Environmental and chemical carcinogenesis. Seminars in Cancer Biology. 2004;**14**(6):473-486

[7] Limoli CL, Giedzinski E, Bonner WM, Cleaver JE. UV-induced replication arrest in the xeroderma pigmentosum variant leads to DNA double-strand breaks, -H2AX formation, and Mre11 relocalization. PNAS. 2002;**99**(1):233-238

[8] Vítor AC, Huertas P, Legube G, de Almeida SF. Studying DNA double-strand break repair: An ever-growing toolbox. Frontiers in Molecular Biosciences. 2020;7:24

[9] Goodenow D, Lalwani K, Richardson C. DNA damage and repair mechanisms triggered by exposure to bioflavonoids and natural compounds. In: DNA-Damages and Repair Mechanisms. London, UK: IntechOpen; 2021. DOI: 10.5772/intechopen.95453

[10] Harper JW, Elledge SJ. The DNA damage response: Ten years after. Molecular Cell. 2007;**28**:739-745

[11] Richardson C, Jasin M. Eukaryotic Recombination: Initiation by Double-strand Breaks. In: Encyclopedia of Life Sciences. Hoboken, New Jersey: John Wiley & Sons, Ltd. 2001;**1**. DOI: 10.1038/npg.els.0000577

[12] Richardson C, Moynahan ME, Jasin M. Double-strand break repair by interchromosomal recombination: Suppression of chromosomal translocations. Genes & Development. 1998;**12**(24):3831-3842. DOI: 10.1101/gad.12.24.3831

[13] Elliott B, Jasin M. Human genome and diseases: Review double-strand breaks and translocations in cancer. Cellular and Molecular Life Sciences. 2001;**59**:373-385

[14] Wiktor-Brown DM, Hendricks CA, Olipitz W, Engelward BP. Age-dependent accumulation of recombinant cells in the mouse pancreas revealed by in situ fluorescence imaging. PNAS. 2006;**103**(32):11862-11867

[15] Tratar UL, Horvat S, Cemazar M. Transgenic mouse models in cancer research. Frontiers in Oncology. 2018;**8**:268

[16] White RR, Milholland B, de Bruin A, Curran S, Laberge RM, van Steeg H, et al. Controlled induction of DNA double-strand breaks in the mouse liver induces features of tissue ageing. Nature Communications. 2015;**6**(1):1-11

[17] Simonatto M, Latella L, Puri PL. DNA damage and cellular differentiation: More questions than responses. Journal of Cellular Physiology. 2007;**213**:642-648

[18] Pandita TK, Richardson C. Chromatin remodeling finds its place in the DNA double-strand break response. Nucleic Acids Research. 2009;**37**(5):1363-1377

[19] Specks J, Nieto-Soler M, Lopez-Contreras AJ, Fernandez-Capetillo O. Modeling the study of DNA damage responses in mice. Methods in Molecular Biology (Clifton, N.J.). 2015;**1267**:413-437

[20] Hakem R. DNA-damage repair; the good, the bad, and the ugly. EMBO Journal. 2008;**27**(4):589-605

[21] Mehta A, Beach A, Haber J. Homology requirements and competition between gene conversion and break-induced replication during double-strand break repair. Molecular Cell. 2017;**65**:515-526

[22] Tubbs A, Nussenzweig A. Endogenous DNA damage as a source of genomic instability in cancer. Cell. 2017;**168**(4):644-656

[23] Coopera TJ, Garcia V, Neale MJ. Meiotic DSB patterning: A multifaceted process. Cell Cycle (Georgetown, Tex). 2016;**15**(1):13-21

[24] Romanienko PJ, Daniel C-OR. The mouse Spo11 gene is required for meiotic chromosome synapsis. Molecular Cell. 2000;**6**:975987

[25] Paiano J, Wu W, Yamada S, Sciascia N, Callen E, Paola Cotrim A, et al. ATM and PRDM9 regulate SPO11-bound recombination intermediates during meiosis. Nature Communications. 2020;**11**:1-15

[26] Jena NR. DNA damage by reactive species: Mechanisms, mutation and repair. Journal of Biosciences. 2012;**37**(3):503-517

[27] Chen CS, Wells PG. Enhanced tumorigenesis in p53 knockout mice exposed in utero to high-dose vitamin E. Carcinogenesis. 2006;**27**(7):1358-1368

[28] Shafirovich V, Kropachev K, Anderson T, Liu Z, Kolbanovskiy M, Martin BD, et al. Base and nucleotide excision repair of oxidatively generated guanine lesions in DNA. Journal of Biological Chemistry. 2016;**291**(10):5309-5319

[29] Marsden CG, Dragon JA, Wallace SS, Sweasy JB. Base excision repair variants in cancer. Methods in Enzymology. 2017;**591**:119-157

[30] Talhaoui I, Matkarimov BT, Tchenio T, Zharkov DO, Saparbaev MK. Aberrant base excision repair pathway of oxidatively damaged DNA: Implications for degenerative diseases. Free Radical Biology and Medicine. 2017;**107**:266-277

[31] Yamtich J, Nemec AA, Keh A, Sweasy JB. Germline polymorphism of DNA polymerase beta induces genomic instability and cellular transformation. PLoS Genetics. 2012;**8**(11):1003052

[32] Zeman MK, Cimprich KA. Causes and consequences of replication stress. Nature Cell Biology. 2014;**16**(1):2

[33] Guirouilh-Barbat J, Lambert S, Bertrand P, Lopez BS, Porro A, Chang M, et al. Is homologous recombination really an error-free process? Frontiers in Genetics. 2014;**5**:175

[34] Wiktor-Brown DM, Olipitz W, Hendricks CA, Rugo RE, Engelward BP. Tissue-specific differences in the accumulation of sequence

rearrangements with age. DNA Repair. 2008;7(5):694-703

[35] Sukup-Jackson MR, Kiraly O, Kay JE, Na L, Rowland EA, Winther KE, et al. Rosa26-GFP direct repeat (RaDR-GFP) mice reveal tissue- and age-dependence of homologous recombination in mammals in vivo. PLoS Genetics. 2014;**10**(6):1-16

[36] Kimoto T, Kay JE, Li N, Engelward BP. Recombinant cells in the lung increase with age via de novo recombination events and clonal expansion. Environmental and Molecular Mutagenesis. 2017;**58**(3):135

[37] Li W, Li F, Huang Q, Shen J, Wolf F, He Y, et al. Quantitative, noninvasive imaging of radiation-induced DNA double-strand breaks in vivo. Cancer Research. 2011;**71**(12):4130-4137

[38] Thompson LH. Recognition, signaling, and repair of DNA double-strand breaks produced by ionizing radiation in mammalian cells: The molecular choreography. Mutation Research—Reviews in Mutation Research. 2012;**751**(2):158-246

[39] Vignard J, Mirey G, Salles B. Ionizing-radiation induced DNA double-strand breaks: A direct and indirect lighting up. Radiotherapy and Oncology. 2013;**108**(3):362-369

[40] Little JB. Genomic instability and bystander effects: A historical perspective. Oncogene. 2003;**22**:6978-6987

[41] Stanley FKT, Berger ND, Pearson DD, Danforth JM, Morrison H, Johnston JE, et al. A high-throughput alpha particle irradiation system for monitoring DNA damage repair, genome instability and screening in human cell and yeast model systems. Nucleic Acids Research. 2020;**48**(19):e111. DOI: 10.1093/nar/gkaa782

[42] Buis J, Wu Y, Deng Y, Leddon J, Westfield G, Eckersdorff M, et al. Mre11 nuclease activity has essential roles in DNA repair and genomic stability distinct from ATM activation. Cell. 2008;**135**(1):85-96

[43] Brodie SG, Xu X, Qiao W, Li W-M, Cao L, Deng C-X. Multiple genetic changes are associated with mammary tumorigenesis in Brca1 conditional knockout mice. Oncogene. 2001;**20**(51):7514-7523

[44] Koike M, Yutoku Y, Koike A. The defect of Ku70 affects sensitivity to X-ray and radiation-induced caspase-dependent apoptosis in lung cells. Journal of Veterinary Medical Science. 2013;**75**(4):415-420

[45] Goff JP, Shields DS, Seki M, Choi S, Epperly MW, Dixon T, et al. Lack of DNA polymerase θ (POLQ) radiosensitizes bone marrow stromal cells in vitro and increases reticulocyte micronuclei after total-body irradiation. Radiation Research. 2009;**172**(2):165-174

[46] Scully R, Panday A, Elango R, Willis NA. DNA double-strand break repair-pathway choice in somatic mammalian cells. Nature Reviews Molecular Cell Biology. 2019;**20**:698-714

[47] Langie SA, Azqueta A, Collins AR. The comet assay: Past, present, and future. Frontiers in Genetics. 2015;**6**:266. DOI: 10.3389/fgene.2015.00266

[48] Kawashima Y, Yamaguchi N, Teshima R, Narahara H, Yamaoka Y, Anai H, et al. Detection of DNA double-strand breaks by pulsed-field gel electrophoresis. Genes to Cells. 2017;**22**(1):84-93

[49] Hayashi M. The micronucleus test-most widely used in vivo genotoxicity test. Genes and Environment. 2016;**38**:18

[50] Kinner A, Wu W, Staudt C, Iliakis G. Gamma-H2AX in recognition and signaling of DNA double-strand breaks in the context of chromatin. Nucleic Acids Research. 2008;**36**:5678-5694

[51] Revet I, Feeney L, Bruguera S, Wilson W, Dong TK, Oh DH, et al. Functional relevance of the histone gammaH2Ax in the response to DNA damaging agents. Proceedings of the National Academy of Sciences of the United States of America. 2011;**108**(21):8663-8667. DOI: 10.1073/pnas.1105866108

[52] Bonner WM, Redon CE, Dickey JS, Nakamura AJ, Sedelnikova OA, Solier S, et al. γH2AX and cancer. Nature Reviews Cancer. 2008;**8**:957-967

[53] Cruz-García A, López-Saavedra A, Huertas P. BRCA1 accelerates CtIP-ediated DNA-end resection. Cell Reports. 2014;**9**(2):451-459

[54] Huertas P, Cruz-García A. Single molecule analysis of resection tracks. Methods in Molecular Biology. Clifton, New Jersey: Humana Press Inc; 2018;**1672**:147-154

[55] Wolf M, Eskerski H, Bauder-Wü St U, Haberkorn U, Eisenhut M. Alkylating benzamides with melanoma cytotoxicity: Experimental chemotherapy in a mouse melanoma model. Melanoma Research. 2006;**16**(6):487-496

[56] Weber GF. DNA damaging drugs. Molecular Therapies of Cancer. 2014;**12**:9-112

[57] Kondo N, Takahashi A, Mori E, Ohnishi K, McKinnon PJ, Sakaki T, et al. DNA ligase IV as a new molecular target for temozolomide. Biochemical and Biophysical Research Communications. 2009;**387**(4):656-660

[58] Galluzzi L, Senovilla L, Vitale I, Michels J, Martins I, Kepp O, et al. Molecular mechanisms of cisplatin resistance. Oncogene. 2012;**31**:1869-1883

[59] Kass EM, Helgadottir HR, Chen CC, Barbera M, Wang R, Westermark UK, et al. Double-strand break repair by homologous recombination in primary mouse somatic cells requires BRCA1 but not the ATM kinase. Proceedings of the National Academy of Sciences of the United States of America. 2013;**110**(14):5564-5569

[60] Hinz JM. Role of homologous recombination in DNA interstrand crosslink repair. Environmental and Molecular Mutagenesis. 2010;**51**:582-603

[61] Nitiss JL, Nitiss KC. Tdp2: A means to fixing the ends. PLoS Genetics. 2013;**9**(3)

[62] Nanya M, Sato M, Tanimoto K, Tozuka M, Mizutani S, Takagi M. Dysregulation of the DNA damage response and KMT2A rearrangement in fetal liver hematopoietic cells. PLoS One. 2015;**10**(12):1-18

[63] Attia SM, Al-Anteet AA, Al-Rasheed NM, Alhaider AA, Al-Harbi MM. Protection of mouse bone marrow from etoposide-induced genomic damage by dexrazoxane. Cancer Chemotherapy and Pharmacology. 2009;**64**(4):837-845

[64] Azarova AM, Lyu YL, Lin CP, Tsai YC, Lau JYN, Wang JC, et al. From the cover: Roles of DNA topoisomerase II isozymes in chemotherapy and secondary malignancies. Proceedings of the National Academy of Sciences of the United States of America. 2007;**104**(26):11014

[65] Meng Z, Qin G, Zhang B. DNA damage in mice treated with sulfur dioxide by inhalation. Environmental and Molecular Mutagenesis. 2005;**46**(3):150-155

[66] Philbrook NA, Winn LM. Benzoquinone toxicity is not prevented by sulforaphane in CD-1 mouse fetal liver cells. Journal of Applied Toxicology. 2016;**36**(8):1015-1024

[67] Tung EWY, Philbrook NA, MacDonald KDD, Winn LM. DNA double-strand breaks and DNA recombination in benzene metabolite-induced genotoxicity. Toxicological Sciences. 2012;**126**(2):569-577

[68] Fenner K, Canonica S, Wackett LP, Elsner M. Evaluating Pesticide Degradation in the Environment: Blind Spots and Emerging Opportunities. Science. 2013;**341**(6147):752-758

[69] Sebastian R, Raghavan SC. Induction of DNA damage and erroneous repair can explain genomic instability caused by endosulfan. Carcinogenesis. 2016;**37**(10):929-940

[70] Bariar B, Vestal CG, Richardson C. Long-term effects of chromatin remodeling and DNA damage in stem cells induced by environmental and dietary agents. Journal of Environmental Pathology, Toxicology and Oncology. 2013;**32**(4):307-327

[71] Ross JA, Kasum CM. Dietary flavonoids: Bioavailability, metabolic effects, and safety. Annual Review of Nutrition. 2002;**22**:19-34

[72] Skibola CF, Smith MT. Potential health impacts of excessive flavonoid intake. Free Radical Biology and Medicine. 2000;**29**(3-4):375-383

[73] Spector LG, Xie Y, Robison LL, Heerema NA, Hilden JM, Lange B, et al. Maternal diet and infant leukemia: The DNA topoisomerase II inhibitor hypothesis: A report from the children's oncology group. Cancer Epidemiology, Biomarkers & Prevention. 2005;**14**(3):651-655. DOI: 10.1158/1055-9965.EPI-04-0602

[74] Schro¨der JP, Schro¨der-Van Der Elst S, van der Heide D, Rokos H, Morreale De Escobar G, Ko¨hrle AJ, et al. Synthetic flavonoids cross the placenta in the rat and are found in fetal brain. The American Journal of Physiology. 1998;**274**(2):E253-E256. DOI: 10.1152/ajpendo.1998.274.2.E253

[75] Strick R, Strissel PL, Borgers S, Smith SL, Rowley JD. Dietary bioflavonoids induce cleavage in the MLL gene and may contribute to infant leukemia. Proceedings of the National Academy of Sciences of the United States of America. 2000;**97**(9):4790-4795. DOI: 10.1073/pnas.070061297

[76] Bariar B, Vestal CG, Deem B, Goodenow D, Ughetta M, Engledove RW, et al. Bioflavonoids promote stable translocations between MLL-AF9 breakpoint cluster regions independent of normal chromosomal context: Model system to screen environmental risks. Environmental and Molecular Mutagenesis. 2019;**60**(2):154-167

[77] Goodenow D, Emmanuel F, Berman C, Sahyouni M, Richardson C. Bioflavonoids cause DNA double-strand breaks and chromosomal translocations through topoisomerase II-dependent and -independent mechanisms. Mutation Research—Genetic Toxicology and Environmental Mutagenesis. 2020;**849**:503144

[78] Vanhees K, Coort S, Ruijters EJB, Godschalk RWL, Schooten FJ, Doorn-Khosrovani SB van W. Epigenetics: Prenatal exposure to genistein

leaves a permanent signature on the hematopoietic lineage. The FASEB Journal. 2011;**25**(2):797-807

[79] Levitsky KL, Toledo-Aral JJ, López-Barneo J, Villadiego J. Direct confocal acquisition of fluorescence from X-gal staining on thick tissue sections. Scientific Reports. 2013;**3**:2937

[80] Gossen J, de Leeuw W. LacZ transgenic mouse models: Their application in genetic toxicology. Mutation Research. 1994;**307**(2):451-459. DOI: 10.1016/0027-5107(94)90256-9

[81] Dean SW, Brooks TM, Burlinson B, Mirsalis J, Myhr B, Recio L, et al. Transgenic mouse mutation assay systems can play an important role in regulatory mutagenicity testing in vivo for the detection of site-of-contact mutagens. Mutagenesis. 1999;**14**(1):141-151. DOI: 10.1093/mutage/14.1.141

[82] Richardson C, Jasin M. Frequent chromosomal translocations induced by DNA double-strand breaks. Nature. 2000;**405**:697-700

[83] Huh WJ, Mysorekar IU, Mills JC. Inducible activation of Cre recombinase in adult mice causes gastric epithelial atrophy, metaplasia, and regenerative changes in the absence of "floxed" alleles. American Journal of Physiology. Gastrointestinal and Liver Physiology. 2010;**299**(2):G368-G380. DOI: 10.1152/ajpgi.00021.2010. Epub 2010 Apr 22

[84] Matos-Rodrigues G, Martini E, Lopez BS. Mouse models for deciphering the impact of homologous recombination on tumorigenesis. Cancers. MDPI AG. 2021;**13**(9):2083

[85] Yang YG, Saidi A, Frappart PO, Min W, Barrucand C, Dumon-Jones V, et al. Conditional deletion of Nbs1 in murine cells reveals its role in branching repair pathways of DNA double-strand breaks. EMBO Journal. 2006;**25**(23):5527-5538

[86] Jasin M. Genetic manipulation of genomes with rare-cutting endonucleases. Trends in Genetics. 1996;**12**(6):224-228

[87] White RR, Sung P, Vestal CG, Benedetto G, Cornelio N, Richardson C. Double-strand break repair by interchromosomal recombination: An in vivo repair mechanism utilized by multiple somatic tissues in mammals. PLoS One. 2013;**8**(12):1-16

[88] Chen CC, Kass EM, Yen WF, Ludwig T, Moynahan ME, Chaudhuri J, et al. ATM loss leads to synthetic lethality in BRCA1 BRCT mutant mice associated with exacerbated defects in homology-directed repair. Proceedings of the National Academy of Sciences of the United States of America. 2017;**114**(29):7665-7670

[89] Vaidya A, Mao Z, Tian X, Spencer B, Seluanov A, Gorbunova V. Knock-in reporter mice demonstrate that DNA repair by non-homologous end joining declines with age. PLoS Genetics. 2014;**10**(7):1-9

[90] Sommer D, Peters AE, Baumgart AK, Beyer M. TALEN-mediated genome engineering to generate targeted mice. Chromosome Research. 2015;**23**(1):43-55

[91] Meyer M, Hrabé De Angelis M, Wurst W, Kühn R. Gene targeting by homologous recombination in mouse zygotes mediated by zinc-finger nucleases. PNAS. 2010;**107**(34):15022-15026. DOI: 10.1073/pnas.1009424107

[92] Doudna JA, Charpentier E. Genome editing. The new frontier of genome engineering with CRISPR-Cas9. Science. 2014;**346**(6213):1258096. DOI: 10.1126/science.1258096

[93] Shin JJ, Schröder MS, Caiado F, Wyman SK, Bray NL, Bordi M, et al. Controlled cycling and quiescence enables efficient HDR in engraftment-enriched adult hematopoietic stem and progenitor cells. Cell Reports. 2020;**32**(9):108093

[94] Botstein D, Chervitz SA, Cherry JM. Yeast as a model organism. Science (New York, N.Y.). 1997;**277**(5330):1259

[95] Zhang B, Tang Z, Li L, Lu LY. NBS1 is required for SPO11-linked DNA double-strand break repair in male meiosis. Cell Death and Differentiation. 2020;**27**(7):2176-2190

[96] Gallardo T, Shirley L, John GB, Castrillon DH. Generation of a germ cell-specific mouse transgenic Cre line. Vasa-Cre. Genesis. 2007;**45**(6):413-417

[97] Mu X, Tu Z, Chen X, Hong Y, Geng Y, Zhang Y, et al. In utero exposure to excessive estrogen impairs homologous recombination and oogenesis via estrogen receptor 2 in mice. Frontiers in Cell and Developmental Biology. 2021;**9**:1352

[98] Donehower LA, Harvey M, Slagle BL, McArthur MJ, Montgomery CA, Butel JS, et al. Mice deficient for p53 are developmentally normal but susceptible to spontaneous tumours. Nature. 1992;**356**(6366):215-221

[99] Hua K, Wang L, Sun J, Zhou N, Zhang Y, Ji F, et al. Impairment of Pol β-related DNA base-excision repair leads to ovarian aging in mice. Aging (Albany NY). 2020;**12**(24):25207-25228

[100] Krishna TH, Mahipal S, Sudhakar A, Sugimoto H, Kalluri R, Rao KS. Reduced DNA gap repair in aging rat neuronal extracts and its restoration by DNA polymerase b and DNA-ligase. Journal of Neurochemistry. 2005;**92**:818-823

Chapter 6

Conditional Mutations and New Genes in Drosophila

Boris F. Chadov and Nina B. Fedorova

Abstract

A new class of mutations of *Drosophila melanogaster* has been generated with the help of γ-irradiation and a new selection procedure; the mutations were named *conditional*. According to the data of genetic analysis, these mutations are discrete regions in DNA but are different from the Mendelian protein-coding genes. The genes associated with these mutations are named *ontogenes*. The general pattern of mutation manifestation matches the pattern characteristic of genetic incompatibility in distant hybridization. Development of monstrosities and the observed meiotic abnormalities suggest that ontogenes control the processes providing the proper spatial cell arrangement and switch-on of protein-coding genes. Ontogenes are active at all stages of the soma's life cycle and germinal tissue. In the character of their manifestation, the ontogenes correspond to the *long noncoding RNAs* in molecular genetics. The developed methods for generating mutant drosophila strains allow the manifestation and population dynamics of the mutants for this important group of genes to be studied.

Keywords: mutagenesis, conditional mutation, ontogene, lncRNA, drosophila

1. Introduction

A living organism is a biological system working under the control of its genetic system. This genetic system is more compact but more intricate in terms of the information content: in addition, it provides ontogenesis and phylogenesis of the organisms. Gregor Mendel founded the way of knowing for both systems: this is the way "from character to gene".

The strategy "from character to gene" has emerged to be true. The examples of the inheritance that follows the Mendelian rules are most numerous. The role of chromosomes and later, the role of DNA in heredity have become clear and the DNA code for the construction of proteins of amino acids was discovered. The Mendelian gene, coding for formation of protein, acquired the status of a universal unit of heredity and, therefore, the basic element of a living organism.

However, full-scale human genome sequencing has shown that the protein-coding genes account for only several percent of the entire genome DNA [1]. This means that genetics has so far studied in detail only a small part of the genome, whereas many fundamentally important characters were omitted. Correspondingly, the concept of the protein-coding gene as a universal basic unit of all living is not completely justified and the existence of other categories of genes cannot be excluded. It is a high time to recall the opinion of Kliment Timiryazev, a prominent biologist, on the second discovery of Mendel's rules. While praising the contribution of Mendel to the understanding of heredity, he warned that the rules for inheritance of alternative characters might appear inapplicable to the inheritance of *some other* characters of an organism [2].

The traits of intraspecific similarity, which are distinguishable in terms of taxonomy of an organism, are among these *other* characteristics. Unlike the Mendelian characters varying within a species, they display no variation. The characters of intraspecific similarity are the particular characters that come to mind when speaking about the functions and structures putatively responsible for the part of the DNA molecule that is not associated with protein-coding genes. As a matter of logic, this larger share should accommodate the genes that are responsible for the conserved characters of a living organism, i.e., the characters of species, genus, class, and so on.

This chapter describes examples of non-Mendelian genes. The classical genetic strategy (from character to gene) has been utilized by the authors in this context as well but with an eye towards the putative existence of the DNA regions with the gene properties distinct from those of Mendelian genes. Hereinafter, the Mendelian genes are regarded as the genes (1) responsible for the formation of alternative characters, (2) inherited in accordance with the Mendel's rules, and (3) coding for proteins.

The detection of a gene according to traditional hybridological procedure consists in of the detection of the variants of the corresponding trait and demonstration of a Mendelian inheritance of the variants. The primary task of the experiments on artificial mutagenesis is to find an individual with a character that distinguishes it from the norm among the offspring of the exposed organism. It is impossible to find the individual carrying a mutation in the gene responsible for a conserved trait since this mutation is a dominant lethal by definition.

As has been theoretically inferred, the lethality of conserved genes is not absolute and the genomes exist where this lethality does not manifest. The procedures searching for the mutations that are dominant lethals in one genome but not dominant lethals in another genome have been designed. The new class of mutations was named *conditional mutations* and the genes responsible for their formation and carrying them, *ontogenes* [3–5]. The name "ontogenes" results from the property of these mutations to form monstrous structures (morphoses).

2. Generation of mutations in ontogenes and maintenance of mutations in culture

2.1 General scheme of approach

By definition, the character is the property in which two objects are similar or different (the categories of similarity and distinction) [6]. The living organisms belonging to the same species carry the characters belonging to both categories. All individuals of a particular species display the characters determining the intraspecific similarity. However, some representatives of a species display the characters determining the intraspecific differences and others do not [3]. The latter category of characters is also known as the *alternative characters.* They are famous for the fact that they allowed Mendel to create his genetic theory of the living.

It is currently known that the characters of intraspecific differences at a genetic level are the variants of protein-coding genes. However, it is yet unclear how the similarity characters are organized in terms of genetics. Undoubtedly, they are also encoded in DNA and most likely represent individual DNA regions (genes); however, their arrangement and function are vague. The issues of the establishment and genetic background of the characters of intraspecific similarity are subject to the genetics of individual development and evolutionary genetics. Although a large toolkit of cytological and molecular methods is available for this these areas, the corresponding solutions are still absent.

The basic information about the characters of intraspecific differences has been obtained in the hybridization experiments currently regarded as classical. The research into the characters of intraspecific similarity could have followed the same path but it has not happened. It was believed that the invariance of the characters made it impossible to conduct genetic analysis by hybridization.

With all the uncertainty of the routes by which the similarity characters have been formed, it is doubtless that they are genetically determined. If so, the similarity in a character means that (1) the genes that determine this character are homozygous, and (2) the emerging mutant alleles are eliminated in heterozygotes. The virtual portrait of a gene responsible for a similarity character is rather specific: *the mutation in a gene is viable in a homozygote but lethal in a heterozygote.* The portrait of a Mendelian gene is opposite: the mutation in a Mendelian gene is viable in a heterozygote but may be lethal in a homozygote [7]. In order to find the genes responsible for similarity, we have searched for the unusual mutations that *would be viable in a homozygote and lethal in heterozygote.*

2.2 Generating mutations in drosophila

Drosophila is a convenient organism for the search for the above-defined mutations. The sons were obtained from the γ-irradiated drosophila females (**Figure 1**); part of these sons presumably carried the target mutation in the X chromosome. As was assumed, the homozygosity for the mutation in the X chromosome (males carry one X chromosome) should guarantee the viability of mutant males. All produced males were individually mated with females; the males that did not give daughters (heterozygotes for the mutation in the X chromosome) were regarded as mutant [8, 9]. The obtained mutations matched the defined requirement, namely, they were viable in males (homozygous for mutation) and lethal in females (heterozygous for mutation).

The main point in this technique is to detect the genes that are lethal in heterozygote (dominant lethals). The first batch of the mutants demonstrated that the dominant lethality of the obtained mutants was *conditional.* This lethality depends not only on the mutation itself but rather of on the genome accommodating this mutation and even on the genome of the mating partner. The mutations were named *conditional* [10] and two additional methods for their generation were proposed. In the first variant, the condition for non-manifestation of a lethal in the chromosome was an inversion in the opposite chromosome [11] and in the second, the condition for non-manifestation of a lethal in the X chromosome was a normal genetic constitution of the mating partner [12]. Once the development of monstrosities was recorded in the mutants, we started to detect the mutants in F_1 according to these monstrosities [13]. Further, having found out that the conditional mutations under permissive genetic conditions are always represented by recessive lethals;, we started to select the target

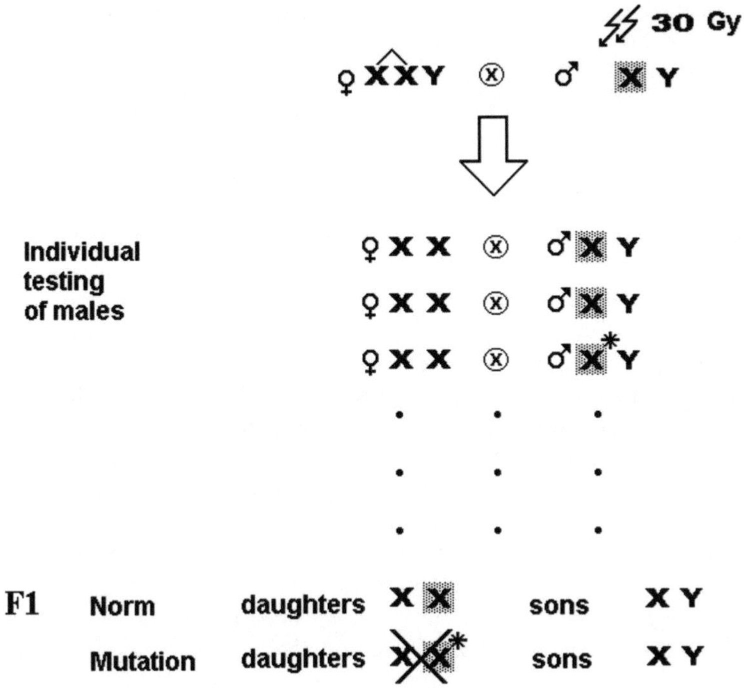

Figure 1.
Detection of conditional dominant lethals in the X chromosome of D. melanogaster. *Gamma-irradiated (30 Gy) Drosophila males were mated to females containing attached-X chromosomes. Sons of this progeny were individually crossed to* yellow *females. X-chromosome of the irradiated male is hatched. Asterisk indicates the same chromosome with mutation. In contrast to sons without lethal mutation, those that received the X with dominant lethal were daughterless.*

mutation from the our collections of recessive lethals [12]. The collection of the drosophila conditional mutations maintained in laboratory at certain times reached a hundred and more variants in the X, 2, and 3 chromosomes.

2.3 Maintenance of conditional mutations in culture

Conditional mutations were maintained in cultures, depending on specificity of each conditional mutation. Conditional dominant lethals in the X chromosome were maintained in two ways (**Figure 2**). With the first way (**Figure 2A**), the culture contained females, heterozygous for the mutation and the Muller-5 inversion. Females produced In (1)M-5 sons and "+" sons with the mutation. The latter were fertile, but no +/+ females appeared in the culture because the effect of the mutation was lethal in the homozygous females. With the second way (**Figure 2B**), the mutant X chromosome was transmitted paternally only so that females in the line contained attached-X chromosomes. Conditional recessive mutations in the X, derived from typical recessive lethals by the Muller-5 method, were maintained as typical recessive lethals in the X chromosome. Conditional dominant lethals in chromosome 2 were maintained in culture containing the In(2LR)Curly inversion. Homozygotes for every one chromosomes 2 were lethal. Conditional dominant lethals in chromosome 3 were maintained in culture containing the In(3LR)Dichaete inversion. Homozygotes for every one chromosomes 3 were lethal.

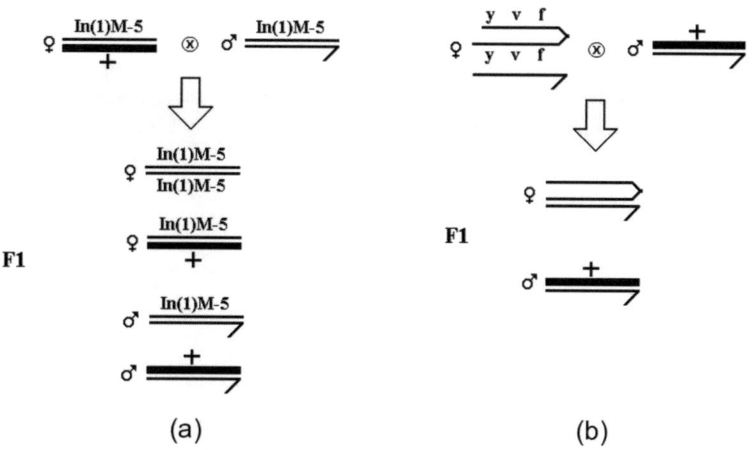

Figure 2.
Two ways for maintenance of conditional dominant mutations in the X chromosome: (a) in heterozygous state in females containing an inverted Muller-5 *chromosome (*In(1) Muller-5*) and the mutant X (+, solid line). Daughters* In(1) Muller-5/+ *and sons + receive the mutant X. Daughters* In(1) Muller-5/In(1) Muller-5 *and sons* In(1) Muller-5 *do not receive the mutant X. (b) in culture with attached-X chromosomes (*y v f/y v f*). Sons, not daughters receive the mutant X chromosome.*

3. Manifestation of mutations in ontogenes

The manifestation of mutations emerged to be numerous and diverse. Some of them are completely unexpected and fantastic, such as the development of monstrosities or changes in the basic metabolism, and others are observable although rarely in common Mendelian mutations (parental inheritance and genetic instability); however, some manifestations are well known for common mutations. The conditional mutations are described in detail in reviews [14, 15]. Here, we give only a brief description to outline these manifestations.

Most of the conditional mutations are dominant lethals. These mutations are characterized by the permissive genetic conditions (genotype) under which a dominant lethal can exist in the organism without leading to its death and the restrictive conditions (genotype) under which its manifests itself. An example is the offspring of the drosophila males carrying a dominant conditional mutation in the X chromosome (**Table 1**). The mutation has no lethal effect in the organism of males but kills the daughters that would form in the crosses of these males with *yellow* females.

In this case, the factor that saves the males from death is their gender (male). In the case of some of the generated dominant conditional mutations, the dominant lethality is eliminated by a chromosome rearrangement in the opposite homolog [11], in a nonhomologous chromosome [12], or even in the genome of the mating partner [12]. The permissive conditions remove the dominant lethality of mutation; however, *recessive lethality* remains so that the homozygotes for mutation die. Recessive lethality under permissive conditions is an obligatory attribute of conditional mutations.

The fact of a recessive lethal manifestation makes it possible to test the mutations for allelism. No alleles have been detected in the large collections of the mutations in the X chromosome (about 60 mutations) and autosome 2 (about 20). The death of mutants in a homozygous state and their survival in a heterozygote with other mutations means that conditional mutations are discrete regions of DNA molecules. Ten conditional mutations in chromosome 2 that displayed recessive lethality were

Mutant male stock no.	Cross: 2♀y x ♂+		Cross: 6♀y x ♂+		Fecundity of male*
	Total number of progenies	Share of daughters in progeny	Total number of progenies	Share of daughters in progeny	
1	119	0.00	191	0.00	0.02
2	650	0.00	435	0.00	0.15
3	112	0.00	180	0.00	0.12
4	114	0.00	293	0.00	0.07
5	50	0.00	303	0.02	0.14
6	47	0.00	283	0.02	0.14
7	47	0.02	100	0.00	—
9	182	0.07	529	0.00	0.40
10	162	0.03	297	0.04	0.09
27	68	0.00	93	0.00	0.18
29	15	0.07	61	0.00	0.14
30	122	0.00	115	0.00	0.19
31	106	0.00	83	0.00	0.15
32	81	0.00	117	0.00	0.13
33	144	0.00	90	0.00	0.16
34	88	0.00	110	0.00	0.12
26	92	0.03	89	0.01	—
35	102	0.03	115	0.04	0.35
36	95	0.00	110	0.01	0.14
37	52	0.02	68	0.04	0.14
38	54	0.06	84	0.01	0.10

**The ratio of adult progenies to the number of laid eggs.*

Table 1.
Progenies and fecundity of mutant (+) males crossed to yellow females [16].

mapped with the help of a standard set of deletions. Half mutants contained two and more lethal defects. These data suggest that the regions of multiple recessive lethality lethalities emerge in a secondary manner under the effect of the earlier formed radiation-induced mutation in ontogene [17].

The conditional mutations with a visible manifestation constitute a separate group. The *Smba* (*Small barrel*) mutation has a dominant phenotype appearing as a shortened body and short pupae. The presence of the *In(2LR)Pm* inversion in the opposite chromosome 2 removed this manifestation. The group of conditional mutations with the phenotypes *scute, radius incompletus,* and *white apricot* manifests only in females, while the corresponding males have a normal phenotype. These mutations were named dimorphic [14].

The permissive genetic conditions allow the dominant lethal mutations in heterozygote to avoid lethality. However, this does not mean that the heterozygotes become completely normal. They have an abnormally high level of locomotor activity and basic metabolism. In addition, they display genetic the instability appearing as (1) activation of the mobile element Dm 412; (2) formation of visible secondary mutations; (3) development of modifications and monstrosities (morphoses); (4) loss of dominant lethal manifestation of mutation with preservation of recessive lethality; and (5) loss of the manifestation of the visible dominant mutations in the chromosome opposite to the mutant homolog [14, 15, 18, 19].

Figures 3 and **4** show examples of modifications and morphoses in the offsprings of mutants. The share of the individuals with morphoses in the offspring of a mutant fly can reach several tens of percent [20, 21]. Because of a strong effect on ontogenesis, the genes responsible for generation of conditional mutations were named *ontogenes* [3–5]. For the sake of brevity, the mutations in ontogenes are hereinafter referred to as *ontomutations.*

A specific feature of ontomutations is that their manifestations are inherited in a parental manner. Thus, the morphoses in a heterozygote for an ontomutation emerge not only in the offsprings that received the ontomutation but also in the offsprings that have not received it [22, 23]. An example of the parental effect is evident for the ontomutations that cause the death of daughters in the crosses with *yellow* females (**Table 1**). The share of dying eggs in the cross is very high (over 50%); this suggests the death not only of the daughters that received the ontomutation, but also of part of the sons that have not received the ontomutation. Meiotic abnormalities hold a special place among all manifestations of ontomutations. This consists in of a high level of chromosome nondisjunction and loss [24] and will be separately considered below.

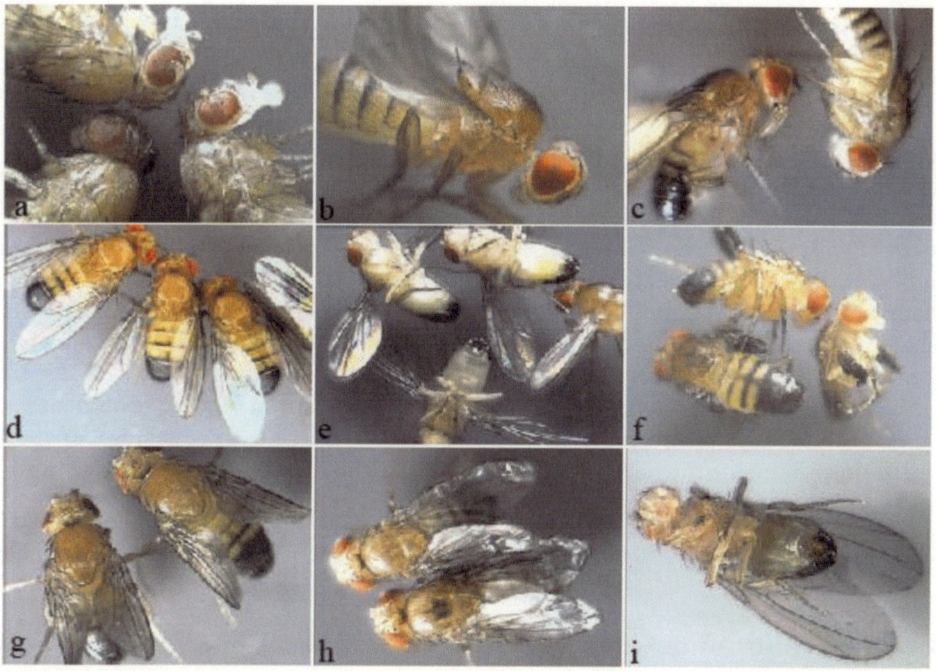

Figure 3.
Modifications in the offspring of conditional mutants: (a) inserted head capsule regions in the eye); (b) a "triangle" eye; (c) defects of the eye shape; (d) narrow wings; (e) pulled apart wings; (f) reduced unspread wings; (g) altered shape of the wings; (h) altered shape of the wings with bubbles and abnormal venation; and (i) interruptions of win veins L4 and L5.

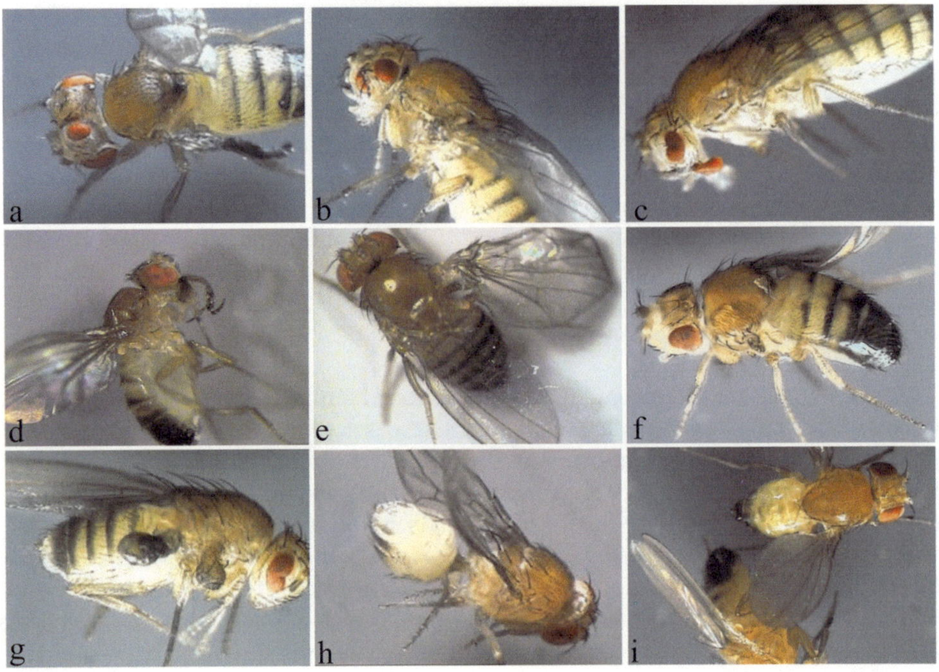

Figure 4.
Morphoses in the offspring of conditional mutants: (a) two heads on one neck; (b) additional head with two eyes instead of the left eye; (c) left eye of two separate fragments; (d) bifurcated tarsus of the right front leg; (e) right wing is widened and contains a bubble; (f) small process instead of the right wing; (g) two processes instead of the right wing; (h) abdomen is turned by 180°; and (i) the upper fly lacks tergites on the abdomen and the right wing is round-shaped.

The pattern of ontomutations manifestations suggests that ontomutations are formed in the genes dissimilar to Mendelian ones. The absence of the own morphological "face" of the majority of ontomutations, the dependence of manifestation on different genetic factors, and the development of morphoses demonstrate that the main function of ontogenes is the regulatory function. However, it has emerged rather difficult in the characterization of ontogenes to advance further than the mere statement of "dissimilarity" and "regulatory character". The range of biological phenomena to be considered and understood appeared to be considerably wider as compared with the Mendelian mutations.

Eventually, it appeared possible to approach the resolution of the question on *the nature of ontogenes,* namely, on what is their biological mission, in which tissues and at which time moments they are active, and what are the forms of this activity. Find below the step-by-step theoretical analysis of the phenomenology of conditional mutations.

4. Manifestation of ontogenes and distant hybridization

Some signs resembling the abnormalities characteristic of distant hybridization were evident in the manifestation of ontomutations. It was reasonable to perform a detailed comparison since a similarity would allow ontogenes to be regarded as the genes responsible for species specificity (membership).

Distant hybridization is the cross of the individual belonging to different taxa (species, genera, families, etc.) [25]. This hybridization is accompanied by the pattern of abnormalities that is independent of a particular cross and of the kingdom to which the parents belong (animals or plants).

The pattern of abnormalities (that is, the pattern of interspecific incompatibility) comprises (1) a high sterility of the cross; (2) parental effect when producing the hybrid; (3) phenotypic mosaicism of the hybrid; and (4) meiotic abnormalities of the hybrid leading to sterility [25, 26]. Characteristic of the ontomutations that we have generated are

1. *Sterility of the cross.* Ontomutations are conditional dominant lethals. The offspring in the crosses of ontomutants can be absent in part or at all. As an example, **Table 2** shows the results of crosses between the strains carrying ontomutations in chromosome 3 [14].

   The males of strain 46 in the crosses with females 34 or 55 give no offspring at all but give offspring with the females of strain 27. The cross of strains 55 and 34 gives no normal offspring but the crosses of mutants of strains 55 and 34 with other strains give normal offspring.

2. *Parental type of inheritance:.* This type of inheritance is a character of the manifestation of ontomutations. **Table 2** clearly demonstrates this effect: two pairs of ontomutations (34 and 46) and (46 and 55) give offspring in one cross direction but do not give it in the opposite direction. Ontomutations display most different forms of the parental effect, both rare in Mendelian mutations or absent at all. This comprises paternal inheritance and paternal–maternal variant

Reciprocal crosses	Progeny						Total number of progeny	*Dichaete* progeny (%)
	Norma			*Dichaete*				
	Females	Males	Total	Females	Males	Total		
♀27 ×♂ 34	49	47	96	20	13	33	129	25.6
♀34 ×♂ 27	56	41	97	114	67	181	278	65.1
♀27 ×♂ 46	132	147	279	34	31	65	344	18.9
♀46 ×♂ 27	63	68	131	102	135	237	368	64.4
♀27 ×♂ 55	88	158	246	29	28	57	303	18.8
♀55 ×♂ 27	37	30	67	97	59	156	223	70.0
♀34 ×♂ 46	0	0	0	0	0	0	0	0
♀46 ×♂ 34	73	95	168	109	95	204	372	54.8
♀46 ×♂ 55	145	166	311	264	279	543	854	63.6
♀55 ×♂ 46	0	0	0	0	0	0	0	0
♀55 ×♂ 34	0	0	0	81	65	146	146	100
♀34 ×♂ 55	0	0	0	114	91	205	205	100

Table 2.
Proportion of Dichaete *progeny in reciprocal crosses of four lines* Dichaete/*mutation [27, 34, 46, 55], containing conditional mutations in chromosome 3.*

[22, 23]. All forms of paternal effects in ontogenes have been described in detail [22, 23, 27].

3. *Mosaicism.* Mosaic fragments are frequently observed in the ontomutants [20, 21]. See **Figure 5** for examples of mosaic phenotypes in ontomutants.

4. *Meiotic abnormalities:.* An extremely high frequency of the X chromosome nondisjunction in meiosis is observed for 30 ontomutations in the drosophila X chromosome [7, 24]. **Table 3** lists the regular and exclusive offsprings of a drosophila female carrying an ontomutation in the X chromosome. The rate of matroclinous daughters (for the X chromosome) reaches 24.7%. In addition to nondisjunction, a loss of the X chromosome is observed and part of the nondisjoined X chromosomes had undergone exchange. A high rate of the X chromosome nondisjunction in drosophila females has a trend of inheritance for the daughters. These data suggest a deep interference into the meiotic division in the ontomutants [24].

As is evident, the pattern of aberrations in the ontomutants is similar to that of the interspecific incompatibility. The question is what the cause of incompatibility is. The heterozygosity in Mendelian genes cannot be the cause of incompatibility because heterozygosity does not lead to lethality in an intraspecific hybridization; moreover, it frequently leads to heterosis. In addition, the mutations in Mendelian genes do not

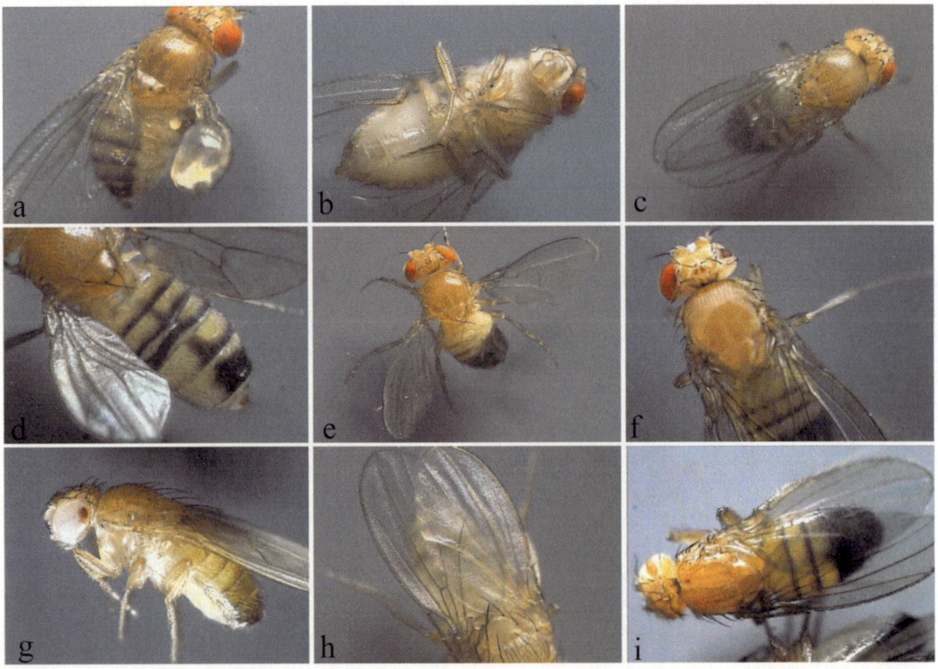

Figure 5.
Mosaics in strains with conditional mutations: (a) the left half of the abdomen is gray the right half, yellow; (b) sex comb is present only on the right front leg; (c) eyes of different colors in the offspring of a w^a*/+ female; (d) colorless left half of last tergites; (e) left half of the abdomen of a female type color and, right, of a male type; (f) different shapes of eyes in the offspring of a B/+ female; (g) as spot of red ommatidia on the background of white ommatidia; (h) yellow left wing and part of the thorax of a gray fly; and (i) right half of the thorax and scutellum are hairless and have no bristles.*

Genotype of female	Regular progeny		Exceptional progeny		Total progeny		Rate of exceptional individuals (%)	
	♀	♂	♀	♂	Imago	With correction to lethality*	♀	♂
l(1)/In(1)	691	380	126	268	1465	2239	11.3	23.9
l(1)/In(1)/Y	373	164	109	154	810	1237	17.6	24.9
l(1)/w	1132	730	362	149	2423	2934	24.7	10.2
w/In(1) (control)	1038	821	10	46	1935	1991	1.0	4.6
w/In(1) (external control 1)	946	922	1	23	1902	1926	0.1	2.4
w/In(1) (external control 2)	842	749	0	20	1638	1658	0	2.4

Table 3.
The effect of mutation in ontogene on the X chromosome nondisjunction in drosophila female meiosis [24].

interfere with meiosis and the corresponding mutants are viable even in compounds with deletion. It is clear that *the heterozygosity in Mendelian genes cannot be responsible for interspecific incompatibility. Correspondingly, the cause underlying the incompatibility is the heterozygosity in the genes that determine the species membership.* In their native genome, these genes are in a homozygous state and thus properly fulfill their role.

The similarity between the manifestations of ontomutations and the pattern of interspecific incompatibility in distant hybridization suggests that (1) the ontogenes belong to the group of the genes responsible for intraspecific similarity and (2) an unusual phenomenology of ontomutations results from their heterozygosity for ontogenes. The latter is similar to the heterozygosity in distant hybridization but is reached in another way. We generate ontomutations with the help of mutagenesis and get heterozygotes for an ontogene by combining them with an initially normal ontogene. Indeed, it is necessary to take into account that all genes responsible for the species membership in an interspecific hybrid are in a heterozygous state versus only one gene (ontogene) in the experiments with ontomutations.

The observed similarity to the pattern of interspecific incompatibility considerably simplifies the understanding of the role of ontogenes in the organism. Any "incompatibility" does not exist for the Mendelian genes and the phenomenon of interspecific incompatibility is determined by the conflict of the genes that form the species specificity of organisms rather than the Mendelian genes. The ontogenes belong to the former group of genes. It is useful to recreate in mind the pattern of incompatibility in distant hybridization to enhance the understanding of the role of ontogenes. Incompatibility is the result of heterozygosity for ontogenes.

5. Ontogenes and construction of cell ensembles

The biological mission of ontogenes was clarified when studying the phenomenon of development of monstrosities (morphoses) in the offspring of an ontomutant (**Figures 6** and 7). In genetic literature, morphosis is defined as a nonadaptive and typically unstable variation of individual morphogenesis associated with a change in the external environment [28–31]. Here, the term morphosis is used to designate the nonheritable morphological abnormalities caused by specific genetic features of the

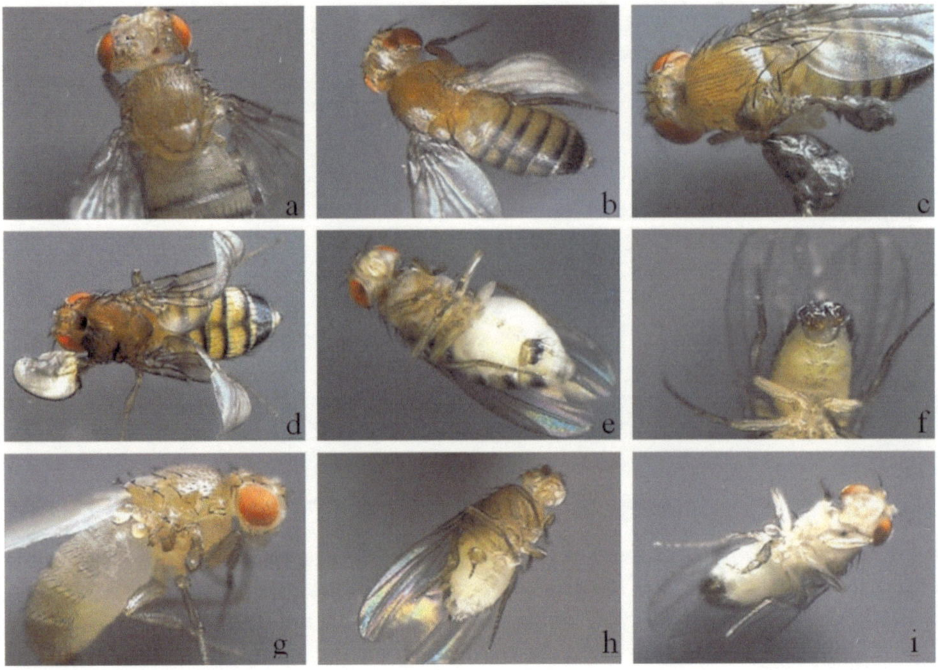

Figure 6.
The morphoses of the "plus tissue" type (surplus structures): (a) groups of eye ommatidia (red spots) on the occiput; (b) an additional eye on the right side; (c) an additional thorax with an altered wing on the right side and a normal wing on the right side in a form of a structure-less bubble; (d) and additional wing on the right side (directed forward) and an altered thorax on the right side; (e) a tergite fragment with bristles on the abdomen; (f) doubling of the external male genitalia; (g) four wing-like appendages with bristles instead of a normal wing on the right side; (h) tarsus on the abdomen; (i) an additional altered seventh leg.

parent itself rather than by the external conditions; correspondingly, they may be referred to as "*endomorphoses*" unlike the earlier known "*exomorphoses*" [21].

The morphoses emerging in conditional mutants are the abnormalities of different degrees of manifestation. Most of them do not prevent flies to hatch from pupae, live, mate, and even give giving offspring. An experimenter working with drosophila for a sufficiently long time has undoubtedly encountered the cases of morphosis development but such cases are very rare. However, morphoses frequently emerge in the offspring of the generated conditional mutants [20, 21]. Soon after commencement of the work with conditional mutations, the collection of colored images of morphoses became very large (about 1000). The diversity and morphological complexity of morphoses are great [32]. The morphological defects are also characteristic of Mendelian mutations but the latter are is incomparably simpler.

The asymmetry of morphoses is the decisive phenomenon in the understanding of the role of ontogenes. *Unlike a bilaterally symmetric morphological defects caused by Mendelian mutations, morphoses are asymmetric:* as a rule, they are present on one side of the body (left or right) [33]. The bilateral asymmetry can be certainly regarded as a cell-level phenomenon. The asymmetry results from an incorrect spatial arrangement of the cells formed by division. Thus, it turns out that ontogenes do control the growth of embryo, its size, and spatial symmetry; moreover, the defects in ontogenes (ontomutations) make asymmetric the normally symmetric structures. The Mendelian genes control production of proteins in cells but do not control the arrangement of

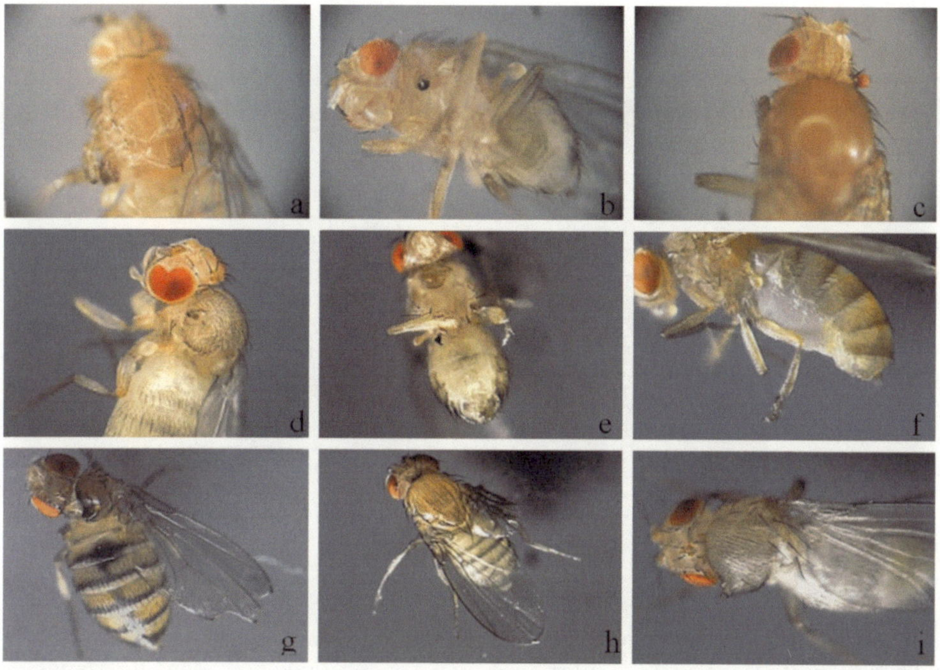

Figure 7.
The morphoses of the "minus tissue" type (lacking morphological structures): (a) loss of a wing (stump) and bristles on the left thorax; (b) loss of a prothoracic leg on the left side; (c) loss of the head cap-sule and major part of the right eye; (d) loss of the left wing and circular bristle pattern on the left thorax; (e) one pair of legs instead of three pairs in the normal fly and different shapes of the right and left legs in the remaining pair; (f) reduced tarsus of the left metathoracic leg; (g) loss of half of the thorax on the left side, including the wing, and a right wing with a Notch-*type indentation; (h) circularly cut right wing; (i) loss of the lift wing and cone-like stretched left thorax.*

cells. That is the reason why Mendelian genes do not interfere with a bilateral symmetry [33].

The involvement of ontogenes in cell spatial arrangement is confirmed by the meiotic abnormalities in ontomutants. As is shown in Section 3, the ontomutations in a heterozygote significantly interfere with the normal meiosis. As is known, the heterozygotes for Mendelian mutations have normal meiosis [34]. Correspondingly, it is reasonable to assert that ontogenes control cell division (in this case, meiotic division) and Mendelian genes do not. Summing up, *the phenomenon of asymmetry of morphoses together with the phenomenon of disturbed meiosis in ontomutants suggests that ontogenes are actually responsible for the construction of cell ensembles.*

It is valid to regard that the "key players" in ontogenesis are now found: they are the ontogenes and Mendelian genes. The former (ontogenes) control the construction of cell ensembles, while the latter controls the production of protein sets in the cells forming the ensembles. To make the picture complete, it is logical to assume that ontogenes also switch on the Mendelian protein-coding genes. The patterns of morphoses in the individuals carrying ontomutations together with mutations in Mendelian genes confirm this assumption.

Consider an example when an additional small head has developed in a fly at the place of the right eye because of a mutation in ontogene (**Figure 8**). Since ontogenes switch on Mendelian genes, the mutant for the Mendelian mutation *Bar* displays the *Bar* phenotype not only for the normal left eye, but also for the aberrant right eye on the newly formed additional small head. It is evident from the available large

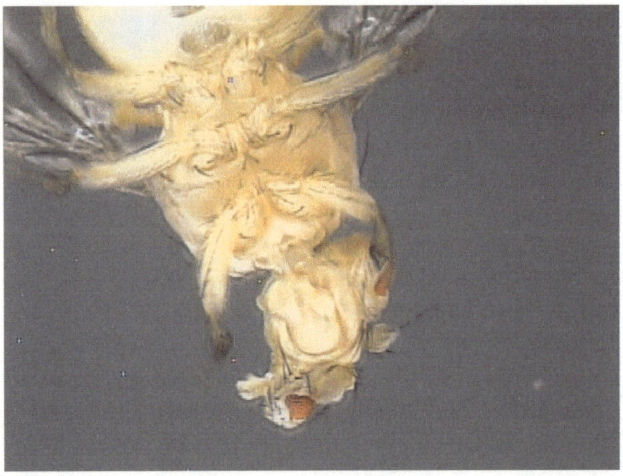

Figure 8.
Morphoses and Mendelian mutation Bar. *Reduced second head in place of the left eye, with the eye on the small head exhibiting a* Bar *phenotype similar to the eye on the main head.*

collection of morphosis images that although the monstrosities are manifold and unusually located, the traits in morphoses that are definitely controlled by Mendelian genes (color of cuticle, eye color, and bristle color) are "switched on" correctly and perfectly fit the fly's genotype. This "adjustment" of the Mendelian genes to the morphological structures despite their pathologies suggests that the event of the switch-on of the structures is automatically the event of the switch-on of a certain set of Mendelian genes.

The discussion of the mechanisms underlying ontogenesis after the works by Jacob and Monod [35] necessarily includes the idea of the regulator genes that trigger the structural genes. It is believed that the regulator genes belong to the category of protein-coding genes. Our data do not contradict the existence of protein regulators but suggest ontogenes as the key players in the organization of ontogenesis. Ontogenesis is not only the production of proteins, but also the *production of the array of cells* housing the production of proteins and ontogenes there are involved in the production of the cell array.

6. Activity of ontogenes in different tissues and at different developmental stages

The Mendelian genes are active in the soma from the very beginning of somatogenesis and to the end of life. According to the experiment, ontogenes are also active in: (1) the germline before meiosis (in premeiosis), (2) during meiotic divisions, and (3) in the zygote at the stage of synkaryon formation.

Premeiosis in germinal tissue:. A half of the offspring of a parent heterozygous for an ontomutation receives the mutation and the other half does not. However, the overwhelming majority of manifestations of ontomutations are observed in the entire offspring. This is true for the emergence of morphoses [22, 23], lethal effect of ontomutations [27], the effect of a chromosome rearrangement on the lethal effect of ontomutation [12, 36], the effect of the Y chromosome on the lethal effect of ontomutation [16], the effect of ontomutation on nondisjunction [24], and so on. All these cases of parental (maternal or paternal) inheritance mean that the mutant ontogenes are active in germline cells. The activity consists in the formation of the "factors" (it is not important which particular factors) that lose a physical link with the ontomutation (DNA region) whereby they originated. As a consequence, these factors after the reduction division equiprobably find themselves in both the gametes carrying ontomutation and the gamete lacking it.

Meiotic division:. Various meiotic abnormalities caused by ontomutations suggest that ontogenes are active in meiosis (see Section 3 and [24] for comprehensive description).

Synkaryon formation. The activity of ontogenes at this stage can be referred to as "the recognition of mating partner" [36]. The *yellow* females do not give daughters in the crosses with the males carrying an ontomutation in the X chromosome (**Table 4**). The prohibition for the presence of daughters in the offspring is removed if the females carry the Cy, Pm, or D inversion in autosomes 2 and 3. It is important that not only the daughters carrying the Cy, Pm, or D autosomes start appearing in the offspring but also the daughters without them. We have assumed that some *tags* appear on the chromosomes of female and male sets during the development of both the female and male gametes of ontomutants as early as the premeiosis. When the chromosome sets enter the zygote, the tags are compared and ontogenesis is triggered in the case the sets display similarity and does not in the absence of similarity [22, 23]. The zygote of drosophila dies at the stage of egg [22, 23]. Formally, this pattern is similar to that when the meeting of pronuclei is prevented, which is observed in genetic incompatibility in plants and protozoans [37, 38].

Male mutation line	Female *y/y*; +/+		Female *y/y*; + / *Cy*				Female *y/y*; + / *Pm*				Female *y/y*; + / *D*			
	Daughter +	Son *y*	Daughter +		Son *y*		Daughter +		Son *y*		Daughter +		Son *y*	
			Cy+	Cy	Cy+	*Cy*	*Pm+*	Pm	*Pm+*	Pm	D^+	*D*	D^+	*D*
1	–	230	–	–	178	163	–	–	107	57	–	–	115	8
2	–	230	14	13	127	134	4	3	70	72	–	–	42	7
4	–	270	9	4	185	159	1	7	86	81	–	–	162	7
5	–	197	23	21	80	95	6	4	47	48	–	–	37	3
27	2	167	1	0	102	113	2	1	53	65	–	–	9	2
29	4	163	32	27	71	56	26	24	55	20	6	6	88	10
30	–	184	15	13	81	76	9	12	60	47	–	–	38	6
31	–	242	32	20	127	102	5	4	28	29	–	–	70	6
32	–	197	22	10	90	77	9	17	36	32	–	–	48	2
33	–	209	20	18	95	101	11	8	87	47	24	2	85	12
34	–	140	11	14	88	101	25	20	68	54	–	10	103	3

Table 4.
Effect of rearranged chromosome 2 and 3 on dominant lethality of conditional mutations in the X chromosome delivered to the zygote together with sperm {cross of mutant males to females: 1) y/y; +/+; *2)* y/y; + / In(2LR)Cy; *3)* y/y; + / In(2LR)Pm *and 4)* y/y; +/ In(3LR) D*} [14].*

Ontogenesis of the soma. The development of morphoses suggests that ontogenes are active at this stage of individual development (see Section 5). A parental type of inheritance of these aberrations [22, 23] indicates that the genetic events in gonial cells are involved in their induction.

As is evident from the list of activities, ontogenes outdo the Mendelian genes in temporal and spatial parameters of their activity. The activity of ontogenes in germinal tissue, where Mendelian genes are inactive, is quite a surprise. The activity of ontogenes at different stages allows for the explanation of an intricate pattern of the ontomutation manifestations. For example, the combination of conditional dominant lethality with definite recessive lethality, illogical at a first glance, is explainable with that the former manifests itself during synkaryon formation and the latter, in the premeiosis of germinal tissue. The activity of ontogenes in the germline for the first time explains the radiation effects appearing as sterility and emergence of mutations in F_1 [39]. The observed activity of ontogenes in the germinal tissue puts the question on the forms of activity of ontogene DNA: a typical form of gene activity is coding for protein synthesis; however, no protein synthesis has been recorded in the germinal tissue.

7. Forms of activity of ontogenes

Activity as nRNA formation.: The chromosome rearrangements of inversion and translocation types interact with ontomutations [12]. The rearrangements themselves act as ontomutations decreasing fertility according to the parental effect [12]. The parental effect suggests the gene activity in the premeiotic cells of the germline. Thus, we may state that a certain chromosome rearrangement in these cells is active and the change in the activity of ontogenes is the result of its presence. Any rearrangement changes the distance between individual ontogenes. If the ontogenes in these cells "communicate" via nRNA, the change in the distances between ontogenes will quite expectedly lead to a change in the function. The lengths of the ways an nRNA have has to cover from an ontogene to another ontogene in a normal genome and in the genome carrying a rearrangement are different. Thus, nRNA can be a regulator of ontogene activity in the premeiotic germline cells.

Usually, proteins act as regulators of gene activity; however, a protein cannot act as a regulator of ontogene activity in germline cells in the case of a rearrangement. The schemes of regulation with the help of a protein and an nRNA are considered in a separate paper [5]. The way of a protein regulator have has to cover in this case (DNA–mRNA–ribosome–protein–DNA) is too long and passes through the cytoplasm. Such regulator will be unable to respond to the minor changes in the distances between ontogenes in the nucleus caused by a rearrangement. On the contrary, an immediate regulation of an ontogene by another ontogene with the help of an nRNA is feasible. All events (synthesis of nRNA and migration of nRNA) and all players (inducer ontogene and receptor ontogene) in this case reside within the nucleus ([5], **Fig. 6**). Thus, the most likely regulators of ontogenes are nuclear noncoding RNAs (ncRNAs). In this case, ontogenes act as both ncRNA inducers and ncRNA recipients.

The recent studies on genome-wide annotation utilizing high-throughput transcriptomics from a single- cell embryo to differentiated tissue cell types demonstrate that over two-thirds of the transcribed mammalian genome codes for tens of thousands of different classes of small and long noncoding RNAs (lncRNAs). The lncRNAs form the largest class of ncRNA subtypes. According to some recent estimates, there exist over 58,084 transcripts in the mammalian genome, which is larger than the number of protein-coding RNAs. In addition, lncRNAs appear to be key regulators in a wide range of biological processes, including cell proliferation, cell cycle, metabolism, apoptosis, differentiation, and pluripotency [40, 41].

It has become clear over the period from generation of the first batch of conditional mutations in *Drosophila melanogaster* in 2000 [8, 9] and a shorter time interval when lncRNA genes were studied [42, 43] that their biological functions are analogous. Both (1) are not protein-coding genes but control the operation of the latter; (2) are elements of the conserved part of the genome; (3) control the progression of ontogenesis and (4) phylogenesis; (5) are responsible for energy exchange in the organism; (6) control cell division; and (7) are inherited according to a parental type. Thus, these two groups most likely represent the same category of genes.

Conformation (coiling and remodeling) of DNA of ontogenes. The fact of a drastic disturbance of cell meiotic division in the presence of an ontomutation has been demonstrated (Section 3). If so, the ontogenes in meiosis are active even taking into account that the chromosomes in a meiotic cell are highly compacted. Thus, the activity is guided by highly compacted DNA of an ontogene and the parental effect on nondisjunction [24] suggests that this coiling "originated" from the premeiotic germline cells.

The previous section discusses the interaction between ontogenes in the zygote, when the parental chromosome sets meet after fertilization [36]. The parental chromosome sets are also highly compacted. The situation there is the same: the ontogenes are active although they are highly compacted. These two facts suggest that *ontogene is a DNA sequence in a state of regulated coiling.* A valid argument favoring this assumption has been earlier obtained by theoretical analysis of the pairing in a heterozygote for inversion [44].

The resulting conclusion focuses the attention on the studies that demonstrate the activity of heterochromatin blocks. Keeping in mind to do this large work in the future, see some studies indicating an important role of heterochromatin in the chromosome behavior in meiosis [45–49]. It cannot be excluded that the multilocality of some ontogenes that we have discovered by deletion mapping of ontomutations in chromosome 2 [17] is explainable with that the ontogenes are represented by coiled repeats. The pattern of somatic pairing in the regions of lncRNAs Firre in different chromosomes suggests the same inference [50].

Biophysical aspect of ontogene activity. The activity of ontogenes coming from compacted chromosome regions suggests that the mutual spatial arrangement of the DNA regions belonging to ontogenes is functionally significant. The studies into the effect of lncRNAs on DNA remodeling [51–53] confirms this. Having commenced the work with mutations in ontogenes, we encountered the cases of interaction of the ontogenes separated by considerable distances [44, 54, 55]. The simplest case is the interaction of the ontogenes that leads to the pairing of homologs in meiosis [44]. Note that the DNA of ontogenes in this process is in a coiled state. It is logical to assume that the forces emerging as a result of coiling of lncRNA regions are the factor that brings the homologs together, however, the mechanism of action of this factor is not clear. The new genes, which undoubtedly exist, fulfill the functions that cannot be implemented by Mendelian genes. Unlike the Mendelian genes, responsible for de novo protein synthesis, ontogenes control the template-based reproduction of DNA molecules as well as the reproduction of the cell itself via its division. In that case, the new genes must possess the capabilities that the Mendelian genes lack. Otherwise, the Mendelian genes themselves could cope with this task.

8. Ontogenes and problems in genetics

Currently, the ontogene, similar to the gene in the early days of genetics, is still hypothetical. The particular solutions will appear in the experiments; however, theoretical studies are also necessary. The specific feature of the moment is in that the concept of ontogene is introduced after a long period when the concept of gene represented by a protein-coding gene variant is a sole (universal) hereditary unit. The possible existence of other kinds of genes besides the Mendelian genes have been asserted by de Vries [56], Filipchenko [57], Timiryazev [2], Timofeev-Ressovsky in his first interpretation of the mutations with a varying manifestation [58], and in the hypothesis by Altukhov and Rychkov on the role of special (unchangeable) genes in speciation [59]. These hypotheses have not been further developed because of "objectlessness": the experimental genetics of that time did not know any other genes except for the Mendelian genes. The discovery of mutations in ontogenes, no matter how "strange" they may be, changes the situation. Theoretical discussion of the genetic problems where the concept of ontogene (or its molecular analog, lncRNA gene) can be utilized seems most important

If we admit the existence of ontogenes, the structure of biological characters becomes universal and simple. Each character comprises (1) the cellular basis and (2) the proteins filling the cells. A Mendelian (simple or monogenic) character is regarded as a virtual structure in which its cellular basis is meant to exist but does not considered, while the protein contained in it is considered. On the contrary, cellular basis of the species-, genus-, family-level, etc. characters is considered but their protein content is omitted.

9. Conclusions

Mutagenesis acts as an architect of the living. Theoretically, only mutations give the possibility to (1) expand the potential of an existing biological species and (2) create new species. Mutations in Mendelian genes actually manage to fulfill the first task but fail in the latter [10, 60]. As has emerged, the problem has a simple solution: in addition to Mendelian genes, the genome contains the genes belonging to another category. Earlier, the mutations putatively belonging to this new category have been generated for drosophila. The new mutations were named conditional and the new genes, ontogenes. Currently, it is most possible that lncRNA genes are the molecular analogs of ontogenes. Here, we attempt to construct the phenomenology of conditional mutations, described earlier, into a logically arranged pattern representing a special part of the genome composed of ontogenes. The work of Mendelian genes on the production of proteins is unfeasible without the ontogenes. The arguments favoring a common nature of ontogenes and lncRNAs are considered in the paper.

The category of genes responsible for the specific outlook of a species is not visible in the case of an intraspecific hybridization but becomes evident in distant hybridization as the syndrome of interspecific incompatibility. The pattern of ontogene manifestation repeats the pattern of interspecific incompatibility. This means that the ontogenes belong to the category of genes that determine the species' specificity. The patterns of monstrosities and meiotic abnormalities reveal the main mission of the ontogenes, namely, the control over construction of cell ensembles in ontogenesis. Concurrently, they also include the Mendelian genes that control protein synthesis.

The ontogenes are active in every living cell in a spatial aspect in the germline and soma and in a temporal aspect, starting from the gonial divisions to the renewal of differentiated somatic cells. Our data suggest us that an event of genome editing, taking place in the premeiosis and involving ontogenes, precedes the formation of every gamete. The specific features in the function of ontogenes underlie the following characteristics untypical of the Mendelian genes: (1) dominant lethal effect; (2) conditional effect; (3) parental inheritance; (4) decrease in fertility; and (5) integral forms of variation referred to as individual and epigenetic variations.

Acknowledgements

The authors thank the Institute of Cytology and Genetics, Siberian Branch, Russian Academy of Sciences, for financial support of this work (budget project no. 0259-2021-0011).

Author details

Boris F. Chadov* and Nina B. Fedorova
Institute of Cytology and Genetics, Russian Academy of Sciences, Novosibirsk, Russian Federation

*Address all correspondence to: boris_chadov@mail.ru

References

[1] Venter J, Adams MD, Myers EW, et al. The sequence of the human genome. Science. 2001;**291**:1304-1351

[2] Timiryazev KA. Collected Works. Vol. 2. Moscow: Sel`khozgiz; 1937-1939. pp. 5-7 [in Russian]

[3] Chadov BF, Chadova EV, Kopyl SA, Artemova EV, Khotskina EA, Fedorova NB. From genetics of intraspecific differences to genetics of intraspecific similarity. Russian Journal of Genetics. 2004;**40**(9):945-958

[4] Chadov BF. Ontogenes in *Drosophila melanogaster*: Genetic features and role in onto – and phylogeny. In: Korogodina VL, Chini A, Durante M, editors. Modern Problems of Genetics, Radiobiology, Radioecology and Evolution. Moscow, Russia: JINR; 2007. pp. 80-91

[5] Fedorova NB, Chadova EV, Chadov BF. Genes and Ontogenes in Drosophila: The Role of RNA Forms. Transcriptomics. 2016;**4**:137. DOI: 10.4172/2329- 8936.1000137

[6] Kondakov NI. Logicheskii slovar–spravochnik (Logical Dictionary–Handbook). Moscow: Nauka; 1975. p. 477

[7] Chadov BF. Mutations capable of inducing speciation. In: Stegnij VN, editor. Evolution Biology. Tomsk: Tomsk State University Press; 2001. pp. 138-162 (in Russian). Available from: http://www.evolbiol.ru

[8] Chadov BF, Chadova EV, Kopyl SA, Fedorova NB. A new class of mutations in Drosophila melanogaster. Doklady Biological Sciences. 2000;**373**:423-426

[9] Chadov BF. Mutations in the regulatory genes in Drosophila melanogaster. In: Proceedings of International Conference on Biodiversity and Dynamics of Ecosystems in North Eurasia; 21–26 August 2000. Novosibirsk: IC@G; 2000. pp. 16-18

[10] Chadov BF. Facultative dominant lethals: Genetics, ontogenesis, and phylogenesis. In: Stegniy VN, editor. Evolutionary Biology. Vol. 2. Tomsk: Tomskogo gosudarstvennogo universiteta; 2002. pp. 118-142 [in Russian]

[11] Chadov BF, Chadova EV, Kopyl SA, Fedorova NB. Delayed activation of the maternal genome during early development of Drosophila. Doklady Biological Sciences. 2001;**378**(1-6): 294-298. DOI: 10.1023/A:1019247615297

[12] Chadov BF, Chadova EV, Khotskina EA, Artemova EV, Fedorova NB. The main effect of chromosomal rearrangement is changing the action of regulatory genes. Russian Journal of Genetics. 2004;**40**(7):723-731. DOI: 10.1023/B:RUGE.0000036520.93159.a5

[13] Fedorova NB, Chadova EV, Khotskina EA, Chadov BF. Conditional mutations: Generation using the technique of morphoses. In: Factors of Experimental Evolution. Collection of Papers. Vol. 8. Kiev: Logos; 2010. pp. 78-83 [in Russian]

[14] Chadov BF, Fedorova NB, Chadova EV, Khotskina EA. Conditional mutations in Drosophila. Journal of Life Sciences. 2011;**5**(3):224-240

[15] Chadov BF, Fedorova NB, Chadova EV. Conditional mutations in Drosophila melanogaster: On the Occasion of the 150th Anniversary of G. Mendel's Report in Brünn. Mutation Research - Reviews in Mutation Research. 2015;**765**:40-55. DOI: 10.1016/j.mrrev.2015.06

[16] Chadov BF. "The image" of the regulatory gene in experiments with Drosophila. Russian Journal of Genetics. 2002;**38**(7):725-734

[17] Chadov BF, Chadova EV, Fedorova NB. Conditional mutations in D. melanogaster: Specific features in localization and secondary mutation. In: Proceedings of the International Conference Chromosoma 2012; 2–7 September 2012. Russia: Novosibirsk; [in Russian]

[18] Chadov BF, Chadova EV, Khotskina EA, Fedorova NB. Conditional lethal mutations shift the genome from stability to instability. Russian Journal of Genetics. 2009;**45**(3):276-286. DOI: 10.1134/S102279540903003X

[19] Fedorova NB, Vasilyeva LA. New evidence of mass induction of transpositions of MGE 412 due to the isogeniszation of forked line of Drosophila. In: Proceedings of the III Congress of the Vavilov Society of Geneticists and Breeders. Genetics in XXI Century: Current State and Prospects of Development; 6-12 June 2004. Vol. 2. Moscow: Genetics Society; 2004. p. 61

[20] Chadov BF, Chadova EV, Kopyl SA, Khotskina EA, Fedorova NB. Genes controlling development: Morphoses, phenocopies, dimorphs and other visible expressions of mutant genes. Russian Journal of Genetics. 2004;**40**(3):271-281. DOI: 10.1023/B%3ARUGE.0000021627.82588.41

[21] Chadov BF, Chadova EV, Fedorova NB. Epigenetic phenomenology in conditional mutants of Drosophila melanogaster: Morphoses and modifications. In: Zakijan SM, Vlasov SM, Dement'eva EV, editors. Epigenetics. Novosibirsk: SD RAN; 2012. pp. 499-533 [in Russian]

[22] Chadov BF, Chadova EV, Fedorova NB. The Genetics of Conditional Mutations and Individual developmental Programs in D. SCIOL Genetics Science. 2017;**1**:3-21. Available from: https://sciol.org/articles/genetic-science/fulltext.php?aid=sgs-1-002

[23] Chadov BF, Chadova EV, Fedorova NB. Conditional mutations in Drosophila: Concept of genes that control individual development. Advances in Bioscience and Biotechnology. 2018;**9**:243-272. DOI: 10.4236/abb.2018.96017

[24] Chadov BF, Fedorova NB. Ontogenes and chromosome nondisjunction in the D. melanogaster meiosis. Advances in Bioscience and Biotechnology. 2021;**12**(1):31-59. DOI: 10.18103/mra.v9i4.2366. Available from: http://www.researchgate

[25] Serebrovsky AS. Animal Hybridization. Moscow–Leningrad: Biomedgiz; 1935. p. 290

[26] Lobashev ME. Distant hybridization. In: Genetics. Leningrad: Leningrad Gosudarstvennogo University; 1967. pp. 491-518 [in Russian]

[27] Chadov BF, Fedorova NB, Chadova EV. Parental effects of conditional mutations and their explanations. Russian Journal of Genetics. 2013;**49**(2):141-150. DOI: 10.1134/S1022795413020038

[28] Rieger R, Michaelis A, Green MM. Glossary of Genetics. Classical and Molecular. Berlin: Springer-Verlag; 1991. p. 553

[29] Frizen G. X-ray morphoses in Drosophila. Biology Zhurnal. 1935;**4**:687-704 [in Russian]

[30] Rapoport IA. Specific morphoses in Drosophila melanogaster caused by chemical compounds. Bulletin of Experimental Biology and Medicine. 1939;**7**:415-417 [in Russian]

[31] Goldschmidt RB, Piternick LK. The genetic background of chemically induced phenocopies in Drosophila. Journal of Experimental Zoology. 1957; **135-136**:127-202-1201-28

[32] Chadov BF, Chadova EV, Fedorova NB. Images of morphoses and modifications in Drosophila melanogaster conditional mutants. Mutation Research/Reviews in Mutation Research. 2015;**765**:40-55. DOI: 10.13140/RG.2.1.2721.9042. Available from: http://www.researchgate

[33] Chadov BF, Fedorova NB. The Mutations Disturbing the Bilateral Symmetry in Drosophila. SCIOL Genetic Science. 2019;**2**:139-152. Available from: https://sciol.org/articles/genetic-science/fulltext.php?aid=sgs-2-015

[34] Chadov BF. Nongomologous chromosome pairing in oogenesis of Drosophila melanogaster. Abstract of dissertation for the degree of Ph.D. Institute of Developmental Biology: Moscow; 1971 [in Russian]

[35] Jacob F, Monod J. Genetic regulatory mechanisms in the synthesis of proteins. Journal of Molecular Biology. 1961;**3**: 318-356

[36] Chadov BF, Chadova EV, Fedorova NB. A Novel Type of Gene Interaction in D. melanogaster. Mutation Research: Fundamental and Molecular Mechanisms of Mutagenesis. 2017;**795**: 27-30. DOI: 10.1016/j.mrfmmm.2017.01.002

[37] Lewis D. Gene-environment interaction: A relationship between dominance, heterosis, phenotypic stability and variability. Heredity. 1954; **8**:333-356

[38] Linskens HF. Physiology der Fortpflanzung and Sexualitat. Fort-schr Botany. 1955;**17**:791-818

[39] Fedorova NB. A mutation in ontogene and radiation-induced instability in Drosophila melanogaster. In: Proceedings of The 5th Congress on Radiation Studies (Radiobiology, Radioecology, and radiation Safety); 10–14 April 2006. Moscow: ICRP. p. 75

[40] Geisler S, Coller J. RNA in unexpected places: Long non-coding RNA functions in diverse cellular contexts. Nature Reviews Molecular Cell Biology. 2013;**14**:699-712

[41] Wang X, Song X, Glass C, Rosenfeld M. The long arm of long noncoding RNAs: Roles as sensors regulating gene transcriptional programs. Cold Spring Harbor Perspectives in Biology. 2010;**3**:a003756-a003756

[42] Akhade VS, Pal D, Kanduri C. Long noncoding RNA: Genome organization and mechanism of action. In: Rao M, editor. Long NonCoding RNA Biology. Advances in Experimental Medicine and Biology. Vol. 1008. Singapore: Springer; 2017. DOI: 10.1007/978-981-10-5203-3_2

[43] Lakhotia SC. From heterochromatin to long noncoding RNAs in Drosophila: Expanding the arena of gene function and regulation. In: Rao M, editor. Long Non Coding RNA Biology. Advances in Experimental Medicine and Biology. Vol. 1008. Singapore: Springer; 2017. DOI: 10.1007/978-981-10-5203-3_3

[44] Chadov BF, Fedorova NB. Ontogenes and the paradox of homologous pairing. Advances in

Bioscience and Biotechnology. 2021;**12**: 1-9. DOI: 10.4236/abb.2021.121001

[45] Chadov BF. Near-centromere heterochromatin and co-orientation of chromosomes in dividing cells of Drosophila. Genetica (Russia). 1987; **23**(6):1082-1087

[46] Chadov BF. Mechanism of chromosome nondisjunction in Drosophila meiosis. In: Abbondandolo A, Vig BK, Roi R, editors. Chromosome Segregation and Aneuploidy-III. Italy. Ispra: E.C. Joint Research Center; 1996. pp. 328-343

[47] Hawley RS et al. There are two mechanisms of achiasmate segregation in Drosophila females, one of which requires heterochromatic homology. Developmental Genetics. 1993;**13**(6): 440-467

[48] Karpen GH, Le MH, Le H. Centric heterochromatin and the efficiency of achiasmate disjunction in Drosophila female meiosis. Science. 1996;**273**(5271): 118-122

[49] Hughes SE et al. Heterochromatic threads connect oscillating chromosomes during prometaphase I in Drosophila oocytes. PLoS Genetics. 2009;**5**(1): e10000348

[50] Hacisuleyman E, Goff L, Trapnell C, et al. Topological organization of multichromosomal regions by the long intergenic noncoding RNA Firre. Nature Structural & Molecular Biology. 2014;**21**: 198-206. DOI: 10.1038/nsmb.2764

[51] Prensner J, Iyer M, Sahu A, Asangani I, Cao Q, Patel L, et al. The long noncoding RNA SChLAP1 promotes aggressive prostate cancer and antagonizes the SWI/SNF complex. Nature Genetics. 2013;**45**:1392-1398

[52] Han P, Li W, Lin C, Yang J, Shang C, Nurnberg S, et al. A long noncoding RNA protects the heart from pathological hypertrophy. Nature. 2014;**514**:102-106

[53] Minajigi A, Froberg J, Wei C, Sunwoo H, Kesner B, Colognori D, et al. A comprehensive Xist interactome reveals cohesin repulsion and an RNA-directed chromosome conformation. Science. 2015;**349**:aab2276

[54] Fedorova NB, Chadov BF. Gene interactions in Drosophila without contacts and chemical intermediaries. In: Abstracts Book of: International Conference on Cell and Experimental Biology (Virtual Conference). 9-11 December 2020. Boston: CEB; 2020. p. 6. Available from: https://cellexpbiol.unitedscientificgroup.org/proceedings/CEB-2020_Abstracts.pdf

[55] Chadov BF, Fedorova NB. Ontogenes and the genetics of intraspecific Similarity. Medical Research Archives. 2021;**9**(4):2-10

[56] Gershenzon CN. Foundations of the modern genetics. Naukova dumka: Kiev; 1983. 220 p [in Russian]

[57] Filipchenko Yu A. The evolutionary idea in biology. Izd. Sobashnikovykh: Moscow; 1923. 287 p [in Russian]

[58] Timofeev-Ressovsky NV. The connection between the gene and external character. In: Gazenko OG, Ivanov VI, editors. Selected Works. Moscow, Meditsina; 1996. pp. 59-84 [in Russian]

[59] Altukhov YP, Rychkov YG. Genetic monomorphism of species and its potential biological significance. Zhurnal Obshchei Biologii. 1972;**33**:281-300 [in Russian]

[60] Chadov BF, Chadova EV, Fedorova NB. Ontogenes and the Problem of Speciation. Journal of Evolutionary Science. 2019;**1**(1):33-47. Available from: https://openaccesspub.org/jes/article/1013